Race, Culture,
and
Mental Disorder

Race, Culture, and Mental Disorder

Philip Rack

Foreword by G. Morris Carstairs

Tavistock Publications
London and New York

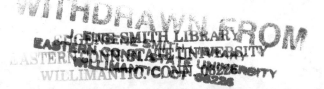

First published in 1982 by
Tavistock Publications Ltd
11 New Fetter Lane, London EC4P 4EE
Published in the USA by
Tavistock Publications
733 Third Avenue, New York, NY 10017

© 1982 Philip Rack

Printed in Great Britain by
J.W. Arrowsmith Ltd., Bristol BS3 2NT

British Library Cataloguing in Publication Data
Rack, Philip
Race, culture, and mental disorder.
1. Mental illness – Diagnosis – Great Britain
2. Minorities – Health and hygiene – Great Britain
I. Title
616.89'075   RC469

ISBN 0–422–781606
ISBN 0–422–781703 Pbk

Library of Congress Cataloguing in Publication Data
Rack, Philip.
Race, culture, and mental disorder.

Includes bibliographical references and indexes.
1. Psychiatry, Transcultural.   2. Personality and
culture.   3. Minorities – Mental health services – Great
Britain.   4. Mental health services – Great Britain.
I. Title.
RC455.4.E8R3 1982   362.2'042   82-10777
ISBN 0–422–78160–6
ISBN 0–422–78170–3 (pbk).

Homo sum; nil a me alienum puto
(Terence, 195–159 BC)

To try to understand the experience of
another it is necessary to dismantle the
world as seen from one's own place within
it, and to reassemble it as seen from his.
(Berger 1975)

Contents

Acknowledgements

In writing this book I received generous support and encouragement from many organizations and individuals. Yorkshire Regional Health Authority allowed me a period of study leave during which I received generous financial support from the Joseph Rowntree Charitable Trust. I am grateful to The British Council for sponsoring a study tour in the Caribbean, and to the Yorkshire Regional Health Authority for support for two visits to Pakistan and India. Two specific research projects were funded by the Commission for Racial Equality and the Yorkshire Regional Research Fund. I am indebted to the Council of MIND, and Charles Clark and Tony Smythe in particular, for practical assistance and advice.

Professor Morris Carstairs, who has kindly contributed the Foreword, has been an unfailing source of guidance for many years.

While I accept sole responsibility for the views expressed here, I must acknowledge how much I have learned from other people, including Professor Henry Murphy in Montreal; Professors Rashid Choudhury and Zaki Hasan, and Dr Laeeq Mirza, in Pakistan; Professors J. S. Neki and Narandra Wig and their colleagues in India; Dr George Mahy and the staff of Black Rock Mental Hospital in Barbados; Drs Frank Knight and Fred Hickling in Jamaica; Dr John Bavington, Mr Nick Farrar, Dr Peter Hitch, and numerous other colleagues in Bradford; Mr Michael Atkins and Ms Susan Atkins; Dr Haru Ghadiali; Ms Marlene Hinshelwood; Ms Jan Webster; and members of the Transcultural Psychiatry Society.

I am grateful to Dr Mohammed Aslam, Mr. Eddie Clarke, Professors Shamai Davidson and Andre Krumperman, and Dr Maurice Lipsedge for allowing me to refer to unpublished work; and to Drs Peter Hitch, Mohammed Aslam and Krishna Vadaddi, Mrs Val Rowell and Ms Pamela Lewis for permission to refer to joint work previously published elsewhere.

In particular I wish to thank my secretaries Mrs Joan Garnett and

Mrs Sheila Fenton for their patient cheerfulness in meeting unreasonable demands; Mr Nick Farrar who read the text and suggested several useful improvements; my friends and colleagues for their support and my family for their tolerance; and above all my patients, from many different cultures, from whom I have learned most of all.

Foreword

The British Isles have long been willing to offer a refuge to individuals and groups who were undergoing persecution in their own countries — provided that they did not come in large numbers. During the Second World War Britain became more than usually multinational because of the influx of soldiery from countries over-run by the Nazis. Belgian, French, Norwegian, and Polish servicemen mixed with companions from America and the Commonwealth. However, it was during the decades which followed that war that we found ourselves, apparently inadvertently, becoming a truly multiracial society thanks to the growing number of immigrants from East and West Africa, from the Caribbean, and from India and Pakistan who came here to work, and to stay. That influx has left us (particularly in London and in the larger industrial cities) with substantial numbers of relatively recent immigrants.

A large proportion of these postwar immigrants were distinguishable not only by their accents or their dress but also by the colour of their skins. They were able to find accommodation and jobs without too much difficulty during the years of full employment; but since the end of the 1960s this has no longer been the case. Having at first been welcomed, especially if they were semi-skilled workers, they now became competitors in a shrinking job market. Immigration began to be a racial problem because some British citizens gave expression to ugly racial prejudices against these recent in-comers. Many other citizens, however, have responded positively by going out of their way in order to help coloured immigrants to become securely integrated.

This book is designed as a source of information about the size and nature of the problem. It starts with a brief history of earlier influxes of immigrants who have been assimilated into the population, and then goes on to describe the cultural characteristics of the major recent groups of incomers. It meets the needs of medical staff, social workers, teachers, and many other people whose work brings them into contact with immigrants to become better informed about the values and customs of these new citizens. Its author, Philip Rack, has been practising as a psychiatrist in Bradford since 1967. Finding himself ill-prepared to understand fully the problems presented by his immigrant patients, he set out to educate himself about their backgrounds and their needs, and he is now sharing the fruits of this self-education with others working in this field. It is not surprising that this initiative has come from Bradford, because nearly 20 per cent of its citizens are immigrants, the majority coming from particular districts of India and Pakistan. Due to Philip Rack's enthusiasm and hard work, his psychiatric unit at Lynfield Mount Hospital in Bradford has become a multidisciplinary centre for the exchange of information and experience between members of all the 'helping professions' whose work brings them in touch with immigrant groups.

Dr Rack does not fall into the trap of thinking that meeting the immigrants' welfare and medical needs are tasks for professionals alone. On the contrary, as an active participant in the local Community Relations Council (of which he has been the Vice-Chairman) he is well aware of the important contributions that can be made both by the immigrants themselves and by members of the host population towards maintaining good relations between the immigrant communities and their British neighbours. He and his wife Anne (a schoolteacher with wide experience of teaching immigrant children) have made friends among the several cultural subcommunities in Bradford. In doing so, he tells us, they have made new discoveries not only about the newcomers, but also about themselves.

This book describes the difficulties that have been encountered by members of these sub-cultures, and how they have been overcome. As a psychiatrist, the author pays special attention to the problems that arise among immigrants, including those who have been refugees. He discusses the need to be aware of cultural beliefs (sometimes of a bizarre and unfamiliar nature) presented by emotionally disturbed immigrants who might erroneously be thought to be suffering from mental illness, and he gives illustrative accounts of the forms in which actual illness, such as manic-depressive psychosis, schizophrenia, hysteria, or psychosomatic disorders are presented by members of particular cultural groups.

On the practical level he describes the recent growth of traditional healing (by Moslem Hakims, Hindu Vaids and West Indian Obeah-men) in several British cities which adds a new exotic dimension to the array of indigenous practitioners of fringe medicine. We are informed about the problems that arise when patients have to be interviewed through the assistance of interpreters; about the different concepts of sickness and of healing; the different expectations of how a doctor should behave which are often brought to the clinical interview; and about the special stresses which can arise within immigrant families when their growing children are exposed to cultural values that contradict some of their parents' deeply held beliefs.

Philip Rack's book can be read with profit by members of the general public — not least, by members of the immigrant communities — and particularly by citizens from any community who wish to be constructively engaged in helping to promote good community relations in their own localities. It is a mine of information for all those who would like to know more about the special problems associated with immigration to this country in recent years, and a source of practical guidance for those who are already engaged in working for (and with) immigrants from a wide variety of cultures.

G. M. CARSTAIRS

Background

Introduction

This book is intended for anyone whose work brings them into contact with members of ethnic minorities. It is about trying to understand unfamiliar problems. The author is a psychiatrist, so much of the contents is derived from experience in dealing with people who are 'mentally ill'. There are sections on the recognition and treatment of mental disorders in different cultures, intended as practical guidance for doctors, nurses, social workers, psychologists, and others whose job it is to offer help when required.

The book is not, however, devoted entirely to clinical matters, because it is impossible to offer help to anyone without understanding their situation, the influences to which they are subjected, and their past and present experiences. We have to take a social and anthropological view as well as a clinical one. We have to take note of beliefs and behaviour which, though unfamiliar, can be understood in social or cultural terms and are *not* evidence of mental disorder.

Mental health specialists deal with only a small fraction of the distress in any community. People do not become psychiatric patients until their mental or emotional problems have become severe. Most people do not become psychiatric patients at all, but everyone experiences stress, and needs the support of family, friends, or others who can help them to overcome difficulties or can show them how to obtain the right sort of help when necessary. In the multicultural society that Britain is today, practitioners in any profession may find themselves trying to help people whose backgrounds are very different from their own.

In a society in which the subject of 'race relations' must be a matter of concern to all thoughtful people, there is an urgent need for better understanding. Those who make policy, those who experience its effects, and those who witness its consequences, should all contribute to the discussion and to the changes which that discussion must produce. But this is not a book about broad social policy, nor does it seek to promote any particular ideology. Basically, it is a book about situations in which two people are facing each other. On one side is a person (or perhaps a family) in some kind of trouble or distress; on the other side is a person (or perhaps a team of people) who want to help. For the sake of convenience we shall refer to the first as the *patient* or *client*, and the second as the *practitioner*; but the practitioner is not necessarily a medical practitioner.

THE PRACTITIONER AND THE CLIENT

In order to provide help, advice, or treatment, the practitioner needs, of course, to know what the problem is, but in the kind of situation we are describing he needs to know more than the immediate facts. He needs to learn the context of the problem and what led up to it, how it appears in the eyes of the client, and the client's reaction to it. He has to get to know the client as a person, and he needs to do these things as expeditiously as possible because his time is limited. When the client is a member of a different ethnic or cultural group, the whole process becomes more difficult.

Irrespective of cultural differences, what the practitioner perceives first is not a *person*, but a *problem*. 'It' is a housing application, a broken arm, an outburst of seemingly crazy behaviour, or a petty larceny. The bearer of the problem is a faceless, indistinct figure. As the conversation or interview gets under way, a picture begins to emerge. The overall shape becomes visible first, followed by increasing detail. The client tries to 'develop' first those details which seem to him most relevant to the immediate problem. The practitioner fills in some of the gaps with direct questions. What started as a two-dimensional outline figure becomes recognizable as a unique individual. The practitioner no longer sees a problem, but a *person with a problem*.

The background of the picture also starts to emerge. The client is not alone: behind him the practitioner glimpses a crowd of other people — family, friends, parents, grandparents, living and dead. Eventually the practitioner can see not a person sitting in a chair talking to him, but a person set in a landscape. It is a distinctive landscape, unique to the individual, though it may contain some familiar landmarks and figures. The practitioner begins to discern some of the milestones and guideposts along the path that the client has trodden to reach his present position, a path that stretches back into the past, into the background of the picture. He may begin to think he can see, more clearly than the client can himself, where the path is leading. In the foreground, the current problem becomes clearer as the circumstances that surround it are more clearly defined. As the picture gains in definition it also gets wider. There is no frame to it, its edges curve round on both sides of the observer like a wide-screen cinema. Crossing some unmarked boundary, the practitioner finds that he is, himself, part of the picture. He is a figure in that landscape, meeting the client at that particular point on the path, interacting with him and with the other figures on it. He has not only identified the problem, but identified *with* the problem. He is, as we say, 'in the picture'.

Described in this way, the process sounds very lengthy and we seem to be crediting the client with considerable descriptive and narrative skill. Of course, many people are quite inarticulate when talking about themselves, and under stress. The practitioner does not get, and probably does not want, a complete view of the whole foreground and background of the landscape. He asks leading questions, flashing a torch on to those areas where he thinks (on the basis of past experience) there may be something relevant. Large blank spaces remain that he does not find it necessary to explore, or that the client seems reluctant to fill in. (If the practitioner is a psychiatrist he will make a note of these.) Most of the background is developed in outline only. Notes such as 'Parents divorced. Father a drunkard. Left home 15. Pregnant at 16. Divorced 20' convey a landscape with which the practitioner is familiar, and if the problem in the foreground also seems to be a recognizable one, that will do for the time being. The practitioner is, in fact, proceeding on the basis of a series of assumptions, generalizations, and associations arising from his previous experience of problems of this kind and his familiarity with this kind of landscape. With a few check questions to test out his impressions, and an ear always open for the unexpected, his assessment is usually adequate. It is incomplete and wrong in some details, but, he hopes, sufficiently accurate where it matters.

This is not the way in which the diagnostic process is taught to students, but it is what happens in practice. The final step, in which the practitioner himself enters the picture, inhabits temporarily the world of his client, and sees it from his standpoint, is in many respects the most important part of the process. The more closely the client's world resembles the practitioner's own world, the more familiar it is, and the more easily is this step taken. But the more different the two worlds, the harder it is to make the identification.

In this book we shall concentrate mainly on situations in which the practitioner is a member of the ethnic majority — probably English by birth, white, and middle-class — and the client or patient is not — probably an immigrant, and often brown or black. The reason for focusing on that situation is quite simply that it is the most common. There are practitioners who are themselves immigrants, or black, or both, but their numbers are relatively small so far, and perhaps they do not need this book.

What are the obstacles that limit the British practitioner's understanding of his ethnic-minority client? If there is no common language the practitioner's picture remains hazy, and may be distorted by verbal ambiguity. The problem might either be a familiar one, expressed in an unfamiliar way, or a completely unfamiliar one: for example, a Muslim father refuses to let his daughter go to school; a woman complains that a neighbour has put a curse on the family; a patient in hospital refuses the prescribed diet. The same behaviour has different meanings in different cultures. An Indian woman who complains of 'gas in the stomach' is trying to convey something rather different from an English woman who say the same thing. An unmarried English girl who becomes pregnant has a problem; so does a Pakistani girl and so does a West Indian girl, but they are not the same problem.

Above all, there is the unfamiliarity of background. The practitioner does not want to know everything about each client, but does want (or *should* want) to locate each figure in its own landscape. If an English client says that his father was a colonel – or a coal-miner; that his childhood was spent in Cheltenham – or Barnsley; these facts do not define the person, but they provide something against which to view him and his present situation. At least, they may indicate some lines of questioning that need *not* be pursued. Moreover, anything that the client says about his father, school, or employment, will probably be couched in terms of which the practitioner can pick up the nuances. But what does it mean if a man was born in Mirpur or Kampala, Barbados or St Kitts? If a West Indian girl was bought up by her grandmother? If a man came to Britain as a European Voluntary Worker? If a client is a Muslim, a Hindu, a Lutheran, a member of the Church of God, or a Rastafarian?

The practitioner is required to enter an unfamiliar landscape where it is not possible to identify important landmarks with a few deft questions, and separate out at a glance the uncommon features from the common ones. To bring the background to life he must painstakingly explore every corner of it. He does not know exactly what he is looking for, and it is an exercise for which he probably has little time or inclination. But the practitioner cannot offer reliable help until he has 'put himself in the picture'. When this process does not happen with an immigrant client, the client remains in the eyes of the practitioner a non-person, a problem thrust forward by an anonymous hand. The difficulties already mentioned, and many others that will be described later, the obstacles to understanding even if there is abundant goodwill, and can be ready-made excuses if there is not.

Faced with these difficulties, we may be tempted to ask: why bother? Why should the busy practitioner go to the trouble of learning about the backgrounds of people who have come to Britain? Surely it is their job to learn our ways, not the other way round? This is an argument to be faced, but it is an argument for the end of the book, after some evidence has been considered, rather than the beginning; and it is, in any case, a theoretical argument. Even if the client *ought* to be forgetting his origins, and even if he will eventually do so, the fact is that at present, at the point of contact, he has not done so, and this is the situation that we as practitioners have to deal with. The cultural background and life experience of such a client influence his habitual responses, reactions to stress, concepts of normality, deviance, and illness, and attitudes to other people — including the practitioner — and it is impossible to deal adequately with such a client without taking those differences into account.

The professional obligation has been well expressed by Roger Ballard:

'For the practitioner the question of whether the minorities ought, or ought not, to remain ethnically distinct should be irrelevant. The fact is that they are. Insofar as his specialism, whatever it is, demands that he should take into account the social and cultural worlds in which his clients live, he needs to make a response to ethnic diversity. If he does not, his practice is inadequate in purely professional terms.'

(Ballard 1979 : 164)

THE NEED FOR CULTURAL UNDERSTANDING

Britain has always been multicultural; there have always been minority groups. Some have come at particular moments in history, either as refugees (e.g. Eastern Europeans, Hungarians, Czechs, Ugandan Asians, Chileans, Vietnamese) or for economic reasons (e.g. Maltese, Cypriots) or a mixture of both. Some have merged into the prevailing culture and disappeared (e.g. Huguenots); others, for example, Jews, have retained a separate identity for many generations. Some — especially those with pigmented skins — are conspicuous and are the subject of much political debate and exaggeration. Others — like the Mauritians and Chinese — seem to pass almost unnoticed.

Even without recent immigrants and their descendants, Britain would be multicultural, containing groups whose lifestyles and beliefs are quite remote from any hypothetical 'norm'. There are differences between social classes, between city and country, between geographical regions, between Catholics and Protestants. Some of these differences are like regional differences in dialect — fascinating in themselves but seldom a serious problem. Others provide fuel for conflict, usually when cultural differences coincide with material inequalities or exploitation.

The cultural differences between social classes, geographical regions, and age-groups are reasonably well documented. Wide gulfs may separate the young, London-trained doctor form the elderly Yorkshire farm-labourer patient, or the middle-class lady magistrate from the fifteen-year-old prostitute, but the territory is fairly well mapped, and once the gulfs are recognized they can be crossed by anyone who has sufficient motivation and sensitivity. But the practitioner facing a Pakistani village woman newly arrived in Bradford, a Nigerian student troubled about black magic, or a frightened Vietnamese refugee, has problems that sensitivity and motivation alone will not solve without real understanding based on knowledge. So it seems better to focus on these newer, more unfamiliar problems — broadly speaking, post-war migrants — and refer to the older, 'internal' differences (important though they are) only when the one can be used to illuminate the other.

We have to try to learn about culture not as an academic exercise, but because in order to understand *why* a person reacts badly to a particular circumstance, one needs to understand what that circumstance meant *to him*, and this is affected by his culture. Different cultures set different boundaries on what is to be regarded as mental illness (rather than some other category of deviant behaviour) and what should be done about it. Whether a client is in the care of a psychiatrist or a probation officer, or both, may depend on the kind of deviance that he displays, which is dependent on his culture, and the response of the society that he is in, which is part of its culture. Furthermore, although it is evident that mental illness exists throughout the world, its manifestations are not everywhere the same. This means that a practitioner working in an unfamiliar culture has to learn some new diagnostic criteria. All these factors must be considered when someone in another culture starts to behave in ways that seem odd, exaggerated, bizarre, or 'ill'. On top of that, when dealing with immigrants, we have to ask how much of the oddness is due to a difference in culture, and how much to being an immigrant in a strange land. If a Nigerian in Britain reacts to stress in ways that seem strange, would his behaviour be recognized as a 'normal' stress reaction in Nigeria? And would there be ways of coping with it by social support, role redefinition, or traditional healing methods, which are not available to him in Britain? If the nature of the stress is not understood, or the way of reacting to it seems strange, there is a danger of being labelled 'ill' or 'mad' unnecessarily, of real illness being missed, or the wrong sort of help given.

Consider, for example, the fairly common situation of the person who believes that he is being persecuted. The complainant is from another culture. He may confide in a doctor, or complain to some authority, or fall into the hands of the police while preparing to defend himself against his persecutors. Before deciding how to approach the problem, we need to know:

(1) Could it be true? Do people in the client's community actually behave to each other in the way being described?
(2) Even if people do not behave like that in Britain, are the client's suspicions explicable in terms of past experiences? (For example, in a concentration camp.)
(3) Even if not that, is the client describing something that is a common *belief* in that community? (Witchcraft, for example, is a common explanation of adversity in many prescientific societies.)
(4) Is it merely a figure of speech, a way of expressing anxiety, not intended to be taken literally?
(5) Is it something in between the last two alternatives? (As in, for example, the apocalyptic imagery of a Rastafarian?)

In this quandary, we need to find signposts wherever we can. There are individual experts, scattered throughout many professions, who have great experience and understanding that is not widely enough shared. We can study clinical descriptions written by practitioners in the countries from which immigrants have come, usually written in English by practitioners who have been trained in our own diagnostic systems, and we may find some who, despite that training, have not lost all contact with the cultures of their countrymen.

A good deal has been written about the behavour of immigrants in general. Britain is not the only country with immigrants, and by taking a broader view we may deduce something about the stresses of the immigration process itself. The sociology of peasants, and of the urbanization process, are studies in themselves. Quite a lot of work has been done on the mental health problems of refugees as a group.

Anthropologists are another useful source of information; but we must not suppose that the culture of a minority group in this country is a microcosm of the country of origin. Cultures evolve continuously, and an immigrant group exposed to new stresses must develop new strategies. Its culture may be somewhere between the traditional one and the surrounding one, but not necessary on a continuum between them — it may well have its own features, derived apparently from neither. To know *this* culture we must recognize its local, transient, and unique characteristics. And *it is only in relation to this culture that we are entitled to say whether or not behaviour is abnormal.*

GENERALIZATIONS AND THE ACCUSATION OF RACISM

As soon as we decide not to judge the normality or deviance of a person's behaviour by comparison with our own cultural norms, but against those of the person's own group, we have taken a step forward, but we are about to fall into a different kind of dilemma. We shall have to try to describe the norms of that group, especially where they differ from our own, and this involves us in making generalizations. Generalizations are at best approximate, and often misleading. Statements such as: 'Immigrants are . . .' 'Black people think . . .', 'Peasants believe . . .', 'The African mentality . . .', 'Muslim attitudes . . .' encourage the formation of those very stereotypes, often with overtones of condescension or criticism, that already bedevil race relations.

People are, of course, much the same all over the world: they are certainly much more the same than they are different. Whether rich or poor, peasant or intellectual, black, white, or any other colour, people have very much the same needs, desires, joys, and sorrows.

> 'Hath not a Jew eyes? Hath not a Jew hands? . . . If you prick us do we not bleed? If you tickle us, do we not laugh? If you poison us, do we not die?'

We have common needs as human beings, and the ways in which we organize ourselves in groups so that those needs can be met within the limits of a particular environment also have a remarkable amount in common. But they are not identical, and even if we were 99 per cent similar and only 1 per cent different, it is the difference that causes the confusion, and it is that small fragment that concerns us at present. It must be emphasized that where differences are noted, we do not have in mind questions of superiority and inferiority. At times we may note that some habitual behaviour is inappropriate in a new environment, or that the strategies adopted by one group seem to be more effective than those of another: but these are not to be construed as statements of the moral worth or fundamental value of the members of those groups. Nor is a difference necessarily a problem. The word 'multicultural' usually occurs in serious discussions about society, often with connotations of worry or concern. We need only substitute the word 'cosmopolitan' to catch the excitement of contrast and variety that should be a stimulus and a delight. Diversity is not usually seen as an asset, but there are signs that this attitude is changing in some places:

> 'all sections of the population have an equal right to the maintenance of their distinctive identities and loyalties of culture, language, religion, and custom . . . their diversity represents an added resource

to the District. The Council will encourage the majority community to realise the full value of this resource and to accept that the minority cultures are an established and lasting component of Bradford's character.'

(City of Bradford Metropolitan Council 1982)

Anthropologists attempt to avoid making external comparisons. They describe a culture *in its own terms* and do not translate concepts, or generalize. This is academically admirable but it leaves us with isolated pockets of knowledge that do not connect up with each other and are not always immediately useful to the practitioner.[1] For the purposes of this book, we are obliged to generalize, to offer propositions about 'migrants' as a class, or 'settlers' as a class, or 'ethnic minorities', or 'Punjabis', or 'peasants', or 'people under stress', or 'psychotic patients', or some other defined group. All such propositions are approximations, and of course it is the case that within any group people act in their own different individual ways. However much we break down our groups into subgroups this must still be true. Whatever we may say about Punjabis in Bradford or Jamaicans in London, we do not expect them all to behave in the way described, nor should we extrapolate too readily to Gujeratis in Leicester or Kittitians in Birmingham. But some extrapolation is justified, and indeed essential. Stereotyping is always undesirable, but generalizations are useful if they help to fill in the background against which an individual can be seen.

Since we are dealing with a subject which arouses strong feelings, it is probably worth adding one further disclaimer. Whenever we point out that in some respect Asians (for example) tend to behave in a manner different from the indigenous British, we may seem to be saying that the British way is normal, and the Asians are peculiar. No such imputation is intended. The British are just as peculiar as anyone else, and their culture is (or, rather, their cultures *are*) distinctive and arbitrary and no more 'right' than any other. But this book is written as a guide for practitioners, not philosophers. A practitioner who sees ten patients in a morning, of whom nine are familiar to him but the tenth is not, wants to know what might be different about the tenth as compared to the other nine. He knows a good deal about the background of the nine, and knows how to obtain whatever information he may lack: the tenth is different. The easiest way for us to describe the difference is by comparison with the other nine. It is not, however, a matter of 'normality' and 'peculiarity'.

NOTES

1   Anthropologists provide immensely useful data, but the practitioner and the anthropologist have different needs and aims. One of the first principles that the student of anthropology learns is that when a group of people is to be described, this must be done as far as possible without preconceptions. The culture is considered and analysed *in its own terms*, not in the terms of the investigator. The practitioner needs to interpret his patient's complaints into terms that he (the practitioner) and his colleagues understand, so that they can fit the problem into a conceptual framework and diagnostic classification (medical or social) for the purpose of providing treatment.

For example, suppose that in a particular tribe two different categories of 'madness' are recognized by the tribe, given different names, and dealt with in different ways. Now it is the case that in contemporary British culture there is also a dichotomy, between *psychosis* and *neurosis*. The anthropologist will not fall into the trap of assuming that the dichotomy in the system used by the tribe is the same as the dichotomy between neurosis and psychosis in his own system. Indeed he will be so much aware of this trap that he will actively avoid it and he may feel that he can only do so by casting out of his mind the psychosis/neurosis dichotomy. His account of any mental illnesses that he observes in his field work will be given in terms of the classification used by that tribe. It is left to the reader to decided how this compares with any other classifications used in other places. Generalizations about a range of groups are not the stock-in-trade of the anthropologist.

The practitioner is in a different position. He has accepted an obligation to offer treatment. He understands his own classification and he uses it because he has found that it works for him (in terms of treatment decisions). He must therefore diagnose his patient in those terms and either ignore the patient's own formulation or find out whether or not it does correlate with his own system. (See, for example, Devereux 1956; Lewis 1971, 1976; Maclean 1971.)

2

Definitions

Britain is frequently described as *multicultural* or *multiracial,* we speak of *ethnic* minorities, and are on the point of changing our *nationality* laws. Do all these terms mean much the same thing?

CULTURE

'Culture' is a term used by anthropologists. A classic definition is: 'that complex whole which includes knowledge, belief, art, morals, law, custom, and any other capabilities and habits acquired by man as a member of society' (Tyler 1874). Leaving aside the definition of belief, art, morals, etc., the important words are 'acquired' and 'as a member of society'. Culture is to do with social conventions. Another definition is:

> 'the categories, plans and rules people use to interpret their world and act purposefully within it . . . the grammar used to construct and interpret behaviour. Culture is learned as children grow up in society. . . . Culture is a plan for behaviour, not behaviour itself.'
> (Spradley and McCurdy 1974 : 2)[1]

Culture is variable and arbitrary. For example, in Britain it is polite to eat with one's mouth closed, in India the opposite.

> 'We tend to think that the norms we follow . . . represent the "natural" way human beings do things. Those who behave otherwise are judged morally wrong, a viewpoint anthropologists consider *ethnocentric*, which means that people think their own culture is the best, or at least the most appropriate way . . . to live.'
> (Spradley and McCurdy 1974 : 3)

Ethnocentrism has powerful emotional reinforcement. Having learned to live by a set of rules, and accepted them unthinkingly during the formative years of childhood, we do not take kindly to having them challenged. Cultures are modified in the face of changes of environment, but alterations tend to be grudging and reluctant. 'One's culture is not like a suit of clothing which can be discarded easily or exchanged for each new lifestyle that comes along. It is rather like a security blanket, and although to some it may appear worn and tattered, outmoded and ridiculous, it has great meaning to its owner'. (Spradley and McCurdy 1974: 5) This is obviously important in relation to cultural dislocation ('culture-shock'), and it may also contribute to the prejudices of the so-called 'host community', since neighbours with a totally different culture, which apparently 'works' fairly well may be a challenge to the comfortable belief that one's own way of life is the only possible one.

Among other things, the rules of behaviour, norms, and customs that constitute culture are an expression of underlying *value systems*. Values are also learned, group-specific, and arbitrary. Some of the values that underlie a culture may strike us as wrong, immoral, and offensive. If, instead of saying that a culture is *bad*, because some of its values are *wrong*, we say this culture is bad and wrong *according to the values of my own culture*, that statement acknowledges that our own values are also culturally determined. This leads us to the proposition known as *cultural relativism*, which may be summarized briefly as:

(1) Each person's value system is a result of his experience, that is, it is learned.
(2) The values that individuals learn differ from one society to another because of different learning experiences.
(3) Values, therefore, are relative to the society in which they occur.
(4) No values are universal: however, we should respect the values of each culture. (Derived from Spradley and McCurdy 1974.)

An older and even simpler statement is: 'There is nothing either good or bad, but thinking makes it so', except that it is not *thinking* that is involved — indeed thinking is usually specifically *not* involved in the formation of value systems, they are accepted without thought. Had Shakespeare been a cultural anthropologist, perhaps Hamlet would have said: 'There is nothing either good or bad but the culturally-determined learned value-systems of a particular society make it so'.

Whether desirable or not, complete cultural relativism is actually impossible: (a) it is internally inconsistent because the proposition that we should respect the values of all cultures is itself a value state-ment; (b) in practice, because no-one can ever escape his own culture and achieve such Olympian detachment; and (c) because it leads to the conclusion that everybody should be allowed to 'do his own thing', which is a denial of social structure and precludes the formation of cultures in the first place. Nonetheless, if we start, as we all do, from a position of ethnocentrism, a large dose of cultural relativism is a useful purgative.

RACE

Race is a biological term. As used by biologists it refers to differences in the inherited, i.e. genetic, constitution of different groups within a species. Man is one species (*homo sapiens*), that much is clear.[2] Within a species, there may or may not be different *breeds* or *races* produced by selective breeding. The differences are extreme in some species (compare a Shire horse with a Shetland pony, or an Alsation with a Pekingese), and comparatively trivial in others. In man, selective breeding came about because of wide geographical separation between different populations, the normal processes of evolution tending to 'reward' those variants that were advantageous in a particular environment, so that the *genetic pool* of a given population tended to contain more of those variants. Races differ to the extent that their genetic pools differ. Individuals within races differ because they draw a different selection of gene-variables (alleles) from the pool. If a particular allele is present in a person's ancestry he may or may not inherit it. If it is not present, he cannot.

On the basis of some of the most obvious physical differences, including skin pigmentation, some geneticists have divided up the species *Man* into races of subspecies (e.g. Caucasian, Mongoloid, Negroid) but there is no universally accepted classification system.[3] An alternative view is that the number of alleles that determine the visible differences between races is such a small proportion of the total genetic constitution that the term 'race' is inappropriate. Proponents of this view claim that when actual allele frequencies have been studied in different so-called races (e.g. 'English', 'Jews', 'Blacks') allele differences are found *within* each group more often than *between* groups. A white American may have European, Asian, African, and Native American components in his ancestry, and might have more genes derived from the Asian or African component, but happen not to have the very small number of alleles responsible for black skin colour. Genetically, Polish Jews have more in common with their non-Jewish neighbours than they do with Spanish Jews. Throughout the European/Asian land mass there has been a persistent movement throughout recorded history from the 'heartlands' of central Asia westward into Europe and southward into India. In both places the preceding inhabitants were 'pushed' towards the end of the peninsula: Celts to the western seaboard of Europe and Dravidians to South India and Sri Lanka. Between those extremes we have a common ('Caucasian') ancestry. Thus, along a line from Britain through Central and Eastern Europe, Ukraine, and eventually to Afghanistan, Pakistan, and North India, there is nowhere a clear demarcation in respect of biological characteristics, each group merges into the next. This kind of continuum is to be found everywhere in the world except where major oceans, deserts, or mountain ranges have prevented travel. Those who engage in disputes as to whether or not races exist within the species *homo sapiens* are merely stating that they do not agree with each other about the meaning of the word race. It is an argument about the relative importance of *within-group differences* and *between-group differences*.[4]

For present purposes it is sufficient to accept that there are some biological differences between different individuals due to their genetic endowment, and that some of these differences occur with greater or lesser frequency in particular groups, which we may or may not choose to call races. The next question is, *does it matter?*

In relation to the behaviour and reactions of any individual, there is no doubt that *culture* is very much more important than *ancestry*. If we have to become involved in a nature-versus-nurture controversy, then certainly nearly all the problems with which practitioners are concerned owe much more to nurture than to nature. But genetically-determined biological variations cannot be overlooked altogether. For example, there are some diseases that have a genetic component and occur only or predominantly among certain geographically-defined groups (e.g. thalassaemia). Also there is some evidence that the metabolic breakdown and de-activation of some drugs is different, so that they are likely to be less effective, or more toxic, in members of certain groups (see Chapter 22).

Second, some geneticists believe that intelligence is related to race. The evidence for this has been hotly disputed, and those who advance it have been castigated as racists. The arguments hinge on the validity of IQ tests, the definition of races, and the technical interpretation of statistics (Montague 1975). The proposition has received little support in Britain, but is still a live issue in some American academic circles, where it is seen as having eugenic consequences. There is even less evidence to support the view that 'personality' or other mental attributes are typical of particular 'races', because such evidence could only be obtained by using tests that had been proved to be 'culture fair' — i.e., free of all possible cultural bias, and no such tests exist.

More important, however, than race as a scientifically valid concept, is the question of race as a social labelling device. This is particularly applicable to people with coloured skins in a predominantly 'white' society. Having said that the most important differences are those of *culture*, it is those to which we shall be paying most attention. However, the differentiation usually applied to immigrants is not in such terms, but in terms of colour. Colour is the greatest single factor which governs society's attitude to members of minority groups and influences their own self-image, and it is inescapable. An Indian or Jamaican in Britain can, if he chooses, abandon the culture of his country of origin, adopt a British life-style completely, and immerse himself totally in his new social environment. He may learn to speak English flawlessly, and if he does not, his children probably will. But neither he nor his children can change their skin colour, and in this respect the coloured immigrant is in a different situation from others — Poles, Ukrainians, Hungarians, Czechs, Maltese, Cypriots, Chileans, and so on — who have preceded or followed him to Britain. We shall need to devote some attention to the social and emotional problems specifically associated with being black.

This introduces another problem of terminology. To refer to all persons who have more pigmentation than the average European as 'black' is quite inaccurate. 'Coloured', is a little less brusque, but there are many immigrants from the northern parts of India or Pakistan whose skin colour is no darker than the average Italian, Spaniard, or Greek — or than an Anglo-Saxon who proudly displays his sun-tan. Are Cypriots or Arabs to be regarded as 'black'?

'From the point of view of the receiving society they may all be lumped together as "coloured people". From the point of view of the different minorities themselves, this is a bizarre terminology, because the different groups have less in common with each other than each of them has with Britain. To the extent that they are treated that way they may come to see themselves as a single group of "coloured people" or "blacks". At present, Asians do not regard themselves as "blacks", and West Indians do not regard themselves as "coloured".' (Smith 1977 : 20)

The practitioner who is aware that coloured people have become understandably sensitive about the way in which white society regards them, will wish to avoid offending sensibilities by using inacceptable terms, and might feel that 'black' is one to avoid. In some circles he will be right: since we have already concluded that culture matters more than colour, it will seem more appropriate to use a cultural term of description. But in other circles, a too-studious avoidance of reference to colour will be criticized as mealy-mouthed doubletalk. The problem is that while some white people have been trying to learn tact, some coloured people have begun to develop a group identity as 'blacks' —

symbolized by the 'Black is Beautiful' slogan — and encourage each
other to wear this badge with pride. One may hear an Indian or Pakistani
speaking about 'us blacks' although his actual complexion is only
marginally different from his 'white' neighbours. He has the right to
proclaim his allegiance, and should not be mocked for doing so. Our
advice to the 'white' practitioner is: (1) it is a matter of courtesy to
treat people on the terms that they themselves propose, at least initially;
but (2) if it is our view that skin colour is not very important, and has
only been made to seem important because people keep mentioning it,
we should not perpetuate this mistake by keeping on mentioning it
unless it is relevant to the specific matter in hand.

A final observation, which summarizes the confusion and absurdity
of 'racial' classification, is that a Pakistani who is 'coloured' or 'black'
in Britain has only to cross the Atlantic to find himself reclassified as
'Caucasian' and therefore 'white'.

ETHNICITY

The term 'ethnic' has come into common use recently, to fill a gap.
Many people are shy of using the word 'race', because they do not
wish to seem to subscribe to beliefs that they do not hold, or because
the term seems to have discreditable associations. But 'culture' has
rather a rather wide set of meanings: we could refer to the cultural
norms of potholers, or ballet dancers. We need a term that indicates
that we are referring to a group with some degree of shared ancestry,
even though we do not consider genetic factors to be very important
determinants of behaviour. 'Ethnic' is a useful word, and at present,
a relatively neutral one.

In this book the terms 'ethnic minority' or 'minority ethnic group'
are used to denote groups that are mainly identified by their culture
(which includes religion) and in which marriage within the group has
been the norm, so that (a) the culture is transmitted from one generation
to the next (though not unchanged), and (b) the group shares a common
genetic pool and members are likely to have heritable as well as cultural
characteristics in common.

In the American literature the usage is different: 'ethnic' is used in
relation to Polish, Italian, Hispanic, or other groups, but not in relation
to black Americans. 'Ethnic studies' and 'Black studies' are different
subjects.

Recently, some sociologists have started to use 'ethnicity' to describe
the processes that hold a group together and maintain its separateness
from the rest of society, the implication being that ethnicity is something
that an individual can either hold on to or abandon according to his choice.

'IMMIGRANT'

Here again there is confusion in terminology, which produces discordant statistics. The numbers of people entering the country are not the same as the numbers entering for settlement, since the former includes students and visitors. Is a person who entered the country thirty years ago and has British citizenship still an immigrant? Does it make a difference if his parents were both British but he happened to be born overseas? There is no easy way through this quicksand and whenever statistics are quoted their precise meaning ought to be explained each time. There is one usage, however, which has no justification and needs to be dropped, and that is 'second-generation immigrant'. We shall use the words 'immigrant' or 'migrant' rather than referring to 'ethnic group', when discussing stresses and other factors connected with the process of migration.

NATIONALITY

Nationality as a concept seems straightforward, but as a matter of law it is very complicated, and British nationality especially so. This is because there are very large numbers of people all over the world who have some kind of relationship with Britain, usually because Britain once ruled their territories or still does. Immigration Acts, passed by successive governments in order to reduce the numbers of people who could claim the right of abode in Britain, have made the position even more complex. Immigration Law is still extremely complex and no attempt will be made here to summarize it since a summary would inevitably be inaccurate. (Specialist advice should be obtained: see Appendix 5.) Nationality Law, however, has been clarified by the *British Nationality Act 1981* which will come into operation in 1982 or 1983. This Act has swept away many anomalies and clarified the legal status of individuals, at the cost of considerable dissatisfaction and some individual injustice.

Under the new Act there will be three categories of citizenship, respectively *British Citizenship, British Dependent Territories Citizenship,* and *British Overseas Citizenship.*

British Citizenship will be granted at the outset to most people who are currently in Britain and have the right of abode here. The right of abode is conferred by virtue of birth, adoption, naturalization, or registration in the UK, or by having a parent or grandparent who was born, adopted, naturalized, or registered in the UK, or through marriage to a man who becomes a British citizen or would have done so but for his death, or through having been legally settled in Britain for five years. After the Act comes into force, British citizenship will be acquired by being born in Britain if one parent is a British citizen but not necessarily otherwise (i.e. in certain circumstances a child born in Britain will not automatically be a British citizen). Children born abroad to British citizens will be British citizens provided that the parent(s) have lived in Britain themselves before that for at least three years, or if a grandparent was a British citizen. If neither condition applies, but the parents subsequently come to live in Britain, the child may apply for registration then. These provisions are clearly intended to set limits to the duration of citizenship by descent in the case of people who although they have citizenship, do not live in Britain.

It will be possible to acquire British citizenship by naturalization. In the case of foreign nationals and Commonwealth citizens, applicants will have to show (as they do now) that they have been resident in Britain for five years and intend to remain, are of good character, and can speak the language. However, in the case of certain people i.e. British Overseas citizens, British Dependent Territories citizens (see below), there is an absolute right of registration as a British citizen after living here for five years. It will also be possible to acquire British citizenship by marriage to a British citizen but not, as in the past, as of right. Apart from some dispensations to cover the period immediately after the Act comes into force, the general principle will be the same for both sexes. The spouse of a British citizen will be admitted for settlement and will be able to apply for naturalization after three years instead of the usual five, provided the marriage has continued. The language qualification will not be applied in such cases.

British Dependent Territories Citizenship applies to persons born in those Territories (which are now few in number) and does not confer automatic right of abode in Britain, except in the case of Gibraltar for which different rules apply under EEC law.[5]

British Overseas Citizenship will be acquired when the Act comes into force by those people who are currently citizens of the United Kingdom and Colonies who do not become British citizens. They will be mainly those whose present citizenship is derived from their residence in a former colony, who opted to retain their British passports at independence. Citizenship will not be transmitted automatically to children born after the Act comes into force, and it does not carry any automatic right of abode in Britain (but see note 5).

It is impossible to predict what problems may arise from the implementation of this Act, in respect of either persons currently resident in Britain or those who may wish to come in future. The numbers of persons admitted for settlement has in any case reduced greatly in rencent years and most of the people who have the right of abode currently will become British citizens when the Act is implemented, by virtue of five years' residence and/or registration. It is claimed that the Act will not affect the position under immigration law of anyone who is lawfully settled in Britain.

NOTES

1 This book of readings provides the non-specialist reader with a useful and readable anthology of contemporary studies in social anthropology. In the past anthropologists usually carried out field work among isolated tribes in remote places, the study of social organization in urban societies being the province of the sociologist. Recently, however, some social anthropologists have turned their attention to urban subcultures, and minority ethnic groups in particular, sometimes combining an account of that group with a study of the environment from which the ethnic group originated. Some recent British examples, to which reference is made in later chapters, are included in Watson (1977) and Saifullah Khan (1979).

2 A *species* is defined by the ability to produce fertile offspring: an ass and a horse can interbreed and produce a mule, but the mule is infertile.

3 Different authors attach importance to different criteria (and this indicates something about their value systems). For example, an American book published in 1978 includes the following table:

Taxonomy of the Living Geographical Races (1)

Subspecies	Trinomen	Alternative Names
Australoid (2)	H. sapiens australicus	Australasid, Australid
Capoid	H. sapiens capitalis	Khoisanid, Khoisan
Caucasoid	H. sapiens caucasus	Europid, Europoid
Mongoloid (3)	H. sapiens asiaticus	Mongolid, Asiatic
Negroid (4)	H. sapiens africanus	Negrid, Congoid

(1) When necessary, hybrid taxa will be denoted as such (e.g. some Afro-Americans, Ainus, Cape Coloureds, Caribbean islanders, Hawaiins, Hottentots, Indo-Dravidians, Indonesians, Melanesians, Mexicans, Polynesians).

(2) Includes several dwarfed local races of Negritos (e.g. parts of India, Southeast Asia, and certain Pacific islands).

(3) Includes numerous local races of Amerinds (North, Central and South America), Aleuts, and Eskimos (circumpolar regions).

(4) Includes dwarfed local races of pygmies (Central Africa).

(from Obsorne, Noble, and Weyl 1978)

The authors introduce this table with the statement that 'Taxonomy is essential for precision in scientific communication'. Unfortunately, they omit to state their criteria for allocation to 'subspecies', 'race', 'local race', 'hybrid', etc. so one only guess at the variables that seem to them to be important.

4   The comparison of *within-group differences* and *between-group differences* is crucial in any system of classification of groups. It can be made to seem very scientific and precise, but sometimes the precision is spurious and the statistics can be manipulated to fit a particular theory. As an example, suppose we had two bags containing coloured marbles, distributed as follows:

	Bag 1	Bag 2	Total
Blue	6	4	10
Green	5	4	10
Yellow	2	8	10
Orange	6	4	10
Red	6	4	10
Total	25	25	

The two bags may be regarded as much the same in respect of their blue, green, orange, and red components, but there is a marked difference in respect of yellow — four times as common in Bag 2 as in Bag 1. A simple statistical calculation will tell us whether the difference is statistically significant, but that only indicates how likely it is to have arisen by chance. Whether the difference is *important* is quite another matter, depending on whether yellow marbles are particularly desirable or undesirable. Supposing that yellow *is* important, we might describe Bag 2 as the yellow-predominating bag, or (since the other variables are roughly equal) the 'yellow bag' for short, and Bag 1 as the 'non-yellow bag'. Now let us suppose that no two marbles are identical in colour: the ones described as green shade off into the blues at one end and the yellows at the other. We might decide to simplify our classification, e.g. by treating the oranges as a variant of red, in which case we have:

	Bag 1	Bag 2	Total
Blue	6	4	10
Green	5	5	10
Yellow	2	8	10
Red (incl. Orange)	12	8	20
Total	25	25	

The proportions remain much the same: the 'yellow bag' still contrasts sharply with the 'non-yellow' one. However, we might have decided to simplify the classification differently, by choosing to regard orange as a variant of yellow.

In that case we get:

	Bag 1	Bag 2	Total
Blue	6	4	10
Green	5	5	10
Yellow Incl. Orange	8	12	20
Red	6	4	10
Total	25	25	

The position is different: there are no longer four times as many yellows in the 'yellow bag' as in the other, the proportion is a mere 3:2 (which in respect of red, blue, etc. we discounted previously). By juggling our within-group differences, we have disposed of the between-group difference. Of course, if our initial distribution had been very unbalanced, it would have been more difficult to manipulate:

	Bag 1	Bag 2	Total
Blue	10	nil	10
Green	6	4	10
Yellow	7	3	10
Orange	2	8	10
Red	nil	10	10
Total	25	25	

This seems like a real and incontrovertible difference. It could be negated, however, by the expedient of redefining blue and red as shades of purple – and stranger things than that have been done in the name of science!

5 In terms of the right of abode in Britain, the only way these two categories of British citizen gain any preference over anyone else is that they have the right of registration after five years' residence.

3

Migration

Before we consider immigration into Britain since 1945, there are three much older population-shifts whose consequences still affect us. Britain used to be a country of *emigration*: in the peak years of 1880–90 a quarter of a million people were leaving *every year* (0.7 per cent of the population) for America, Australia, and other distant destinations (Johnson 1966). This outflow was itself a consequence of a longer process, lasting from the sixteenth to the nineteenth centuries, in which Europeans dominated vast areas of other continents by a system of conquest and settlement that we call the colonial era, and others call white imperialism. That outburst of energy had effects that seem to be permanent in the temperate zones (the Americas, South Africa, and Australasia) but temporary and now coming to an end elsewhere. Several important legacies remain: one is the tangled mess of British nationality and citizenship laws; another is the assumption of superiority by the 'white races'.

Another important mass migration was the slave trade, in which at least ten and perhaps fifteen million people were transported across the Atlantic from West Africa to America and the Caribbean Islands (Franklin 1966). White Britons may choose to regard this as ancient history, but to many black Americans and West Indians it is as significant as the holocaust is to Jews.

Like it or not, attitudes in Britain and attitudes to the British are influenced by history.

RECENT IMMIGRANTS TO BRITAIN

Jews

The ethnic diversity of British did not originate in Jamaica or the Punjab in the 1960s, but in Russia in 1881, for that was the year in which the Pogroms reached their peak. Between 1870 and 1914 about three million Jews fled from Russia and Eastern Europe. America was the ultimate goal for most, but at least 120,000 got no further than Britain. There had of course been Jews in Britain previously. They were deported following 'race riots' in the thirteenth century, but returned in the sixteenth century, fugitives from the Inquisition in Spain and Portugal. Those sophisticated and often wealthy *Sephardic* Jews were followed later by the *Ashkenazi* from Eastern Europe who were often poor and relatively unskilled Yiddish speakers, more strict in their religious orthodoxy. But the refugees who arrived in the 1880s were poorer still, dispossessed peasants who arrived destitute of money or mercantile know-how. They settled in the poorest parts of East London, Manchester, and Leeds in what are now traditional immigrant quarters, and they were the first group to receive the full force of British xenophobia. In the 1930s, as in the 1980s, unemployment and economic recession were the harbingers of racial hatred, and inner-city squalor was its arena. The battle of Cable Street — still within living memory — was the forerunner of post-war confrontations and the origin of the Public Order Act that is still invoked to control them. The National Front is still as anti-semitic as it is anti-black. Despite all this, Jews have prospered, and they come low down the statistics of crime, mental illness, and alcoholism. No-one seems to know why this is so, but the factors usually mentioned include family support and cohesion, firm religious convictions, and rigorous discipline imposed by the group on the individual and by the individual on himself. No-one can say how long Jews will retain their ethnic identity: there are many Jews in the present generation who do not base their sense of identity on their Jewishness, and mixed marriages are becoming more common.

Irish

There is no immigration control between Britian and Eire, so regular statistics are not available, but the 1971 census showed 709,235 Eire-born residents in Britain, amounting to 1.4 per cent of the total population. Many of these are migrant workers (see below) who have no intention of remaining permanently in Britain but retain their roots back home, and this group includes a predominance of single men engaged in unskilled or casual employment. Cheap Irish labour has been a feature of English economic life since the eighteenth century, and their ranks were swelled by refugees from the potato famine, so that by 1861 one quarter of the population of Liverpool was Irish-born. Not all people of Irish ancestry are migrant workers, therefore; there is a large permanent and settled population (notably in Glasgow and Liverpool). But between these two extremes there is a group of whom it is probably fair to say they have roots in neither country, and that might correlate with the observation that the Irish have the highest incidence of mental illness of all immigrant groups. (Cochrane 1977; see also Bagley and Binitie 1970; Clare 1974).

Post-war refugees

'When the victorious Allied Armies appeared in Central Euope, they found approximately nine million displaced persons and prisoners of war living in camps or as billeted forced labourers. The great majority of these people had looked forward to the day when they could rejoin their families at home . . . and by the end of 1945 some 6½ million had done so. But while those from Western Europe had returned to a man, many of those from Eastern Europe were showing considerable hesitation.'   (Tannahill 1958 : 20 3)

These people who preferred to remain on the Western side of the Iron Curtain, included nationals of the Baltic States (Estonia, Latvia, and Lithuania); Byelorussia and the Ukraine; Poland, Czechoslovakia, Yugoslavia, and other parts of Eastern Europe and the Balkans.

At this time Britain, like the other victorious nations, needed labour for reconstruction work. From 1947 officials from the Ministry of Labour toured the Displaced Persons Camps in Europe, and the so-called 'European Volunteer Workers' were induced to come to Britain. They were allowed to 'work their passage to British Citizenship' by filling the vacancies in certain specified jobs (especially agriculture and coal-mining for the men, and textile industries for the women). By December 1950, their numbers in Britain were 85,363, of whom the largest single group were Polish. There were also 94,000 Polish ex-servicemen in Britain, soon joined by 32,000 relatives, bringing the total population of Polish nationals alone to a peak of 157,000. Emigration to America reduced the number to 120,000 by 1954 (Tannahill 1958).

Poles in particular enjoyed some public goodwill as wartime allies. Voluntary and Government agencies were set up to meet their specific needs, and the Polish Resettlement Act of 1947 established three Polish hospitals, special hostels, National Assistance, education grants, and facilities which were by no means commonplace in those early days of the Welfare State. But even during the war there had been some expressions of hostility by sections of the media, and in 1946–47 British xenophobia had reasserted itself, with the familiar accusations that the foreigners were living in luxury at the taxpayer's expense, or alternatively were flooding the labour market and causing unemployment, and were sexually rapacious, morally unscrupulous, cryptofascists, or papist spies (Zubkzycki 1956; Tannahill 1958).

All social and professional classes were represented among these exiles. After completing their compulsory stints in mining or agriculture they took what jobs were available and began the slow process of social and economic advancement. They tended to move to centres of labour-intensive industry (e.g. textiles, engineering) where unskilled work could be obtained despite lack of fluency in English, and in those centres local communities of Poles, Ukrainians, Lithuanians, and others sprang up, often with their own club, church, and social organization — many of which still exist. The original exiles still have a tendency to live near one another and keep in touch and there are deliberate attempts to maintain a separate ethnicity through language classes for the children, dance groups, and social gatherings, but many of the younger generation dismiss these as irrelevant exercises in nostalgia and opt for a lifestyle indistinguishable from the British, to the disappointment of their parents.

There are significant cultural differences between Poland (and different areas within Poland), Lithuania, Latvia, Estonia, Byelorussia, and Ukraine, and different languages. Patriotism remains strong for the older generation, and they do not take kindly to being lumped together as 'Eastern Europeans' or Russians. Poles may react negatively if addressed in either Russian or German. Some Ukrainians (from the Western or 'European' end of the country) speak Polish and have a similar culture to the Poles: those from the Eastern parts are more likely to speak Ukrainian (which is a separate language) or Russian. Polish immigrants seem to be particularly vulnerable to mental break-down, and particularly to paranoia (see Chapter 13).

Hungarian refugees

The Hungarian uprising in 1956 and its suppression caused the next exodus of refugees to the West. This group included a large proportion of young men, and a study at the time (Mezey 1960a, 1960b) suggested that many were restless or rootless individuals, socially and perhaps emotionally unstable, in no way typical of Hungarians as a whole or refugees as a group. Those who have remained in Britain seem to have been assimilated into the community. There are no large Hungarian enclaves, and there does not appear to have been any systematic follow-up to Mezey's initial research.

West Indians

The West Indies has been over-populated, and therefore an emigration area, for generations, many West Indians having gone to America until

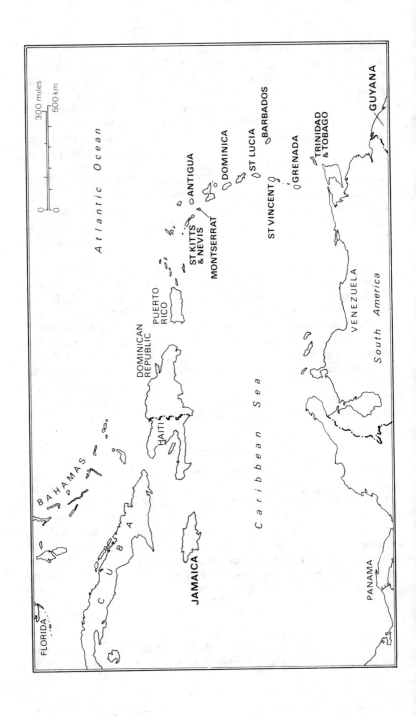

this was curtailed by the McCarran Act 1952. A few had come to Britain during the war, but it was the arrival of 500 Jamaicans in 1948 on the s.s. Windrush that marked the beginning of large-scale Caribbean migration to Britain and the beginning of 'colour' as a factor in British social and political life. Until 1962 there were no restrictions on commonwealth citizens entering Britain, and during the 1950s Britain had a continuing need for labour, especially in low-paid and unskilled jobs. Public organizations like London Transport adopted a policy of overseas recruitment, and some private firms did the same. By 1968, 320,000 West Indians had come to Britain. The proportions of men to women were about 52:40. They were mostly young, and they came to work. They did not necessarily intend to stay permanently, but they expected to be able to fit easily into British society because they had been taught to regard Britain as the 'mother country'. (See Chapter 13, p. 137). They settled in those cities where work was available, and the numbers arriving were an accurate reflection of the fluctuations in the labour market, year by year and even quarter by quarter. The largest number came from Jamaica, but all the Commonwealth Caribbean islands and Guyana were represented. Each is different: there is no 'typical West Indian'. Jamaica is almost the size of Wales and contains a city (Kingston) and several large towns. Ever since obtaining political independence from Britain, Jamaica has been beset by economic problems. There is a good deal of urban squalor and social unrest. Other West Indians say that Jamaicans are hard, aggressive, and pushy — stereotypes not unlike those inflicted on Geordies or Glaswegians in Britain. Granada, St Vincent, St Lucia, Dominica, Antigua, Montserrat, St Kitts/Nevis, Barbuda, and Anguilla are all small islands less than thirty miles across, in which most of the population live in coastal fishing villages or one main town. Life moves at a slow pace, and standards of living and literacy tend to be low. Jamaicans say that 'Small Islanders' are sleepy and parochial. Barbados is different again, being relatively flat, fertile, and intensively cultivated throughout. Although the whole island is densely populated there is relatively little serious poverty and few slums. Compared to the other Caribbean islands, Barbados has an air of settled respectability reminiscent of one of the sleepier English shires. There is universal secondary education, a University campus, and relatively advanced public services and hospitals. Barbadians regard themselves as intellectually a cut above their neighbours.

The West Indian immigrants of the 1950s were not uneducated simpletons capable of dull manual work and nothing else — even if some of their employers chose to think of them that way. Dominica, for example, is not the most technically advanced of the islands; but of six thousand emigrants from Dominica between 1955 and 1960, 1,642 were skilled workers (carpenters, masons, mechanics, etc.), and 118 were qualified professionals (Royer 1977). According to Royer one of the motives for emigration was possessing a skill and being unable to make sufficient headway in a limited environment. A person who was in one job at the age of eighteen had a 75 per cent chance of being in the same job at the age of fifty. Although the main motive for migration was always economic, other factors included a wish to 'see the world' and to get away from the sometimes claustrophobic atmosphere of a small community. Royer comments that in a small island it is impossible to be anonymous, or to conceal one's personal history or day-to-day experiences.

In some cases families travelled together, but more often a man would come on his own, and if he was already married he might send for his wife and family later. This has to be understood in the context of West Indian family structure, which is slightly different from the European pattern (see Chapter 7). All overseas migrants, whether in America, Canada, Britain, or elsewhere, were expected to send regular remittances for the support of their families back home (Lowenthal 1972; Foner 1977).

Indians and Pakistanis

The Indian subcontinent was governed by Britain until 1948. It was an amalgamation of territories with varying degrees of autonomy, and marked cultural differences between regions. At independence the subcontinent was partitioned, those states that were predominantly Hindu and Sikh became India, and those that were predominantly Muslim became Pakistan. (See map.) At the time of partition the religious minorities which were on the 'wrong side' could migrate across. In the Punjab, which was split down the middle, Hindus in the western part fled east, while Muslims in the east went westward, and these movements were accompanied by a great deal of bloodshed. There are still many Muslims in India, but very few Hindus or Sikhs in Pakistan. The corporate nationhood of Pakistan depends heavily on Islam. Apart from religion, East and West Pakistan never had a great deal in common, and East Pakistan eventually became the independent country of Bangla Desh. Relations between India and Pakistan have been strained since 1948. Both countries have experienced internal political instability and there is widespread and severe poverty in both, and population pressure in rural and urban areas. There has been a continuing dispute about Kashmir, which both countries claim.

There is a long tradition of emigration from the villages of Punjab,

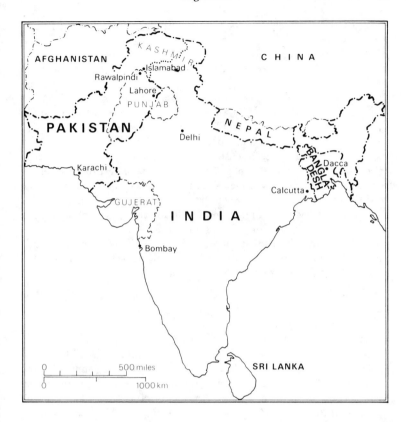

Kashmir, and Bangla Desh. Punjab and Kashmir were favourite recruiting grounds for the army in the days of the Raj, and Bengal provided many merchant seamen on British ships (there were pre-war settlements in British ports of Bengalis who had jumped ship). Post-war migration to Britain started a little later than West Indian migration and reached its peak in the 1960s. They came for the same reason — to find work — and initially by invitation. There are Indian and Pakistani immigrants in other countries, including Scandinavia and Canada, but there is a feeling of affinity to Britain for historical reasons, and some feel that Britain has a special responsibility for the socio-economic problems that make emigration necessary.

The first arrivals in Britain were almost entirely young men. They sent home money and good news, and were soon joined by others from the same family or village, who settled in the same cities, forming particular ethnic enclaves. They took jobs that the indigenous British did not want, and the reaction of the host community was initially neither friendly nor unfriendly, but indifferent. Later, the economic climate deteriorated. Some immigrants had started to exercise their right to bring wives and children to join them, and the presence of fairly large numbers of dark-skinned people in certain cities, living in a style that the British found strange, and competing for a diminishing number of jobs, aroused hostile comment. From 1962 a series of increasingly restrictive immigration laws were passed. This legislation had a paradoxical effect: sensing that the door was closing, people tried to get in before it slammed. The increase in applications (especially for the wives and families of men already here) exacerbated the anxieties of those British who saw their country being 'swamped by alien hordes'. Since 1973 it has been almost impossible for any 'new' immigrants to enter, and the numbers of relatives admitted have also diminished. But still the public believes that there are 'many millions' of coloured immigrants in the country, whereas the real figure (1971 census) is 1.8 million, about 3.3 per cent of the population.

Cypriots

During the post-war years there was a steady migration of Cypriots to Britain and in 1966 the Cypriot population, including children, was estimated as 100,000. After 1962 the numbers admitted annually were reduced to a trickle, except that during the Greek/Turkish conflict in 1974–75 several thousands were admitted as refugees. Unlike the other groups already mentioned, the Cypriot migration included a large number of small families with young children, as well as young men on their own. They tended to settle in London and have established a high degree of economic autonomy based initially on the catering trade but later diversifying into other small businesses. Cypriot family life is centred on the nuclear unit of parents and children, but wider kinship obligations are recognized and there is a good deal of mutual aid within the community, and strong ties with relatives still in Cyprus (Ladbury 1977; Oakley 1979; Constantinides 1977).

West Africans

According to 1971 census figures there were over 46,000 people resident in Britain who were born in West Africa, and that may have been an understimate. The majority were, in some sense, students. In a survey carried out in London:

'66% of the men said that they had come to England in order to get professional or technical qualifications . . . many had succeeded in obtaining necessary preliminary qualifications . . . and in entering degree courses or specialist professional and technical courses . . . some had completed these and were waiting to return home . . . only two per cent planned to remain here permanently.'

(Goody and Groothues 1977 : 154, 164)

For many, however, studentship had been interrupted or prolonged by the need to earn money and support a family at the same time, and some admitted that they were 'not very *serious* students' or not able to study full-time as they would have wished. Goody and Groothues reported that three-quarters of their sample had been in Britain for six or more years, and 40 per cent for more than eight years. Since that study was completed, Government action has drastically increased the fees that Universities must charge overseas students (see also Copeland 1968).

Recent refugees

Significant numbers of Czechs came to Britain in 1968, East African Asians were expelled from Uganda in 1972, Chileans and Argentinians since 1974, and Vietnamese in 1979–80. (See Chapter 16 on refugees in general.)

It is important to differentiate between the 'African Asians' and the Punjabis and other Asians who came to Britain 'direct'. Whereas many of the latter have come from villages in the more remote and under-developed parts of their country, the Kenyan and Ugandan Asians had been prosperous middle-class merchants enjoying a high standard of urban living, often highly educated and literate in more than one language. Many had relatives already in Britain, or in India, Canada, or elsewhere, and their traditional Hindu family culture had been already modified to some extent by a cosmopolitan outlook.

Migrant workers

The term 'migrant worker' is reserved for those who are admitted for a limited period, to take up particular employment, and if they leave that employment they are supposed to leave the country immediately. This is the pattern of *Gastarbeiter* mobile labour in Germany and other European industrial countries, but it operates in Britain on a small scale only. A work permit has to be obtained by the prospective employers, who must show that they have been unable to recruit a suitable worker from the resident workforce. In the past, work permits were issued for domestic servants, workers in the hotel/catering industry, and hospital auxiliaries, and their holders include Spanish, Portuguese, Morroccan, and Filipino nationals; but the quotas have been reduced year by year. Certain professions, of which medicine is one, are exempt from work permits, but the government could withdraw this exemption, and might do so if there were sufficient 'home-produced' doctors available.

MOTIVES FOR MIGRATION

The diversity of the groups listed above makes it quite apparent that generalizations about 'immigrants' are crude and inappropriate. We have to specify according to country (or culture) of origin and reason for coming. Sociologists have proposed various systems of classification (Petersen 1958; Jackson 1969; and review in Anwar 1979) of which the simplest is the 'Pull-factor/Push-factor' distinction. (Did they come because positively attracted to the new country, or to escape from the old? (Patterson 1963).) For our purposes a useful distinction seems to be between *Gastarbeiters*, settlers, and exiles. The distinction is not absolute, and an individual may be in an ambiguous position, or move from one to another: that does not invalidate the classification – on the contrary, we shall argue that it illuminates some of the psychological stresses.

Gastarbeiters

The German word (which means migrant worker) is used because the term Migrant Worker has specific legal meanings (see above) and we are concerned here with attitudes rather than legal status. *Gastarbeiter* migration is a consequence of industrialization, and the movement is generally from rural to urban environements. The pull of the cities is greatest for people in the most undeveloped rural areas because there is no work at home. This is, of course, a well-known historical tendency, likened to 'the tendency of water to flow uphill, when forced by machinery' (Hardy 1891). The industrial centres of Germany, France, Switzerland, Belgium, and Luxemburg attracted workers from the rural periphery of Spain, Portugal, Algeria, Morocco, Southern Italy, Greece, Yugoslavia, and Turkey. In 1976 there were about 15 million foreign workers in industrial Western Europe. Switzerland alone employed one million, accounting for 25 per cent of the labour force. As Spaniards moved northward, Moroccans moved into Spain.

Gastarbeiters are disposable labour. When the economy goes into recession, they can be sent back to where they came from. Voices are raised:

> 'demanding that they go home and leave what jobs there are for home-grown workers . . . In Switzerland the throwing-out is official. No Swiss national can be laid off unless the foreign workers have already been dismissed . . . In West Germany, priority . . . is given to nationals. The children of immigrant workers . . . who may well have spent most of their lives in West Germany, find it difficult to get work permits . . . In the United States . . . because many immigrants' presence is clandestine, the unemployed among them are, through force of circumstances, shifted back home to base. . . . In France . . . The North African and Portuguese immigrants call it to the policy of the lemon: first you squeeze the fruit and then you throw it away . . . After years of economic growth with low-cost service in the engine room provided by non-demanding hard-working immigrants governments now wish they would go home.'
>
> (Power and Hardman 1976 : 37)

Harsh as this is, it is a situation to which the *Gastarbeiter* has himself contributed. When he set out, he never intended to remain permanently in the industrial country to which he went. Commonly a young man goes abroad on his own, leaving his family behind. As much of his earnings as possible are sent home as remittances for the support of his family and to be banked against his return. His long-term aim is to improve his economic and social position back home, and to this end he is prepared to work long hours and live as cheaply as possible. He is not highly motivated to learn about the surrounding culture or to acquire any more of the language than is necessary for survival. He prefers to live with fellow-countrymen, and he is not disposed to modify his habits except to avoid trouble. His emotional roots are in his country of origin. To expect this young man to 'integrate', or criticize him for holding on to his culture, is to miss the whole point of his operation.

Settlers

Unlike *Gastarbeiters*, settlers arrive in the new country with the intention of making their homes there permanently. They tend, therefore, to consist of young families or young married couples with adventurous or innovative ideas, whose ambitions are (they feel) thwarted at home. The massive transatlantic migrations of the nineteenth century were a desperate escape from poverty. For post-war settlers the issues were less stark, but the intention was basically the same: a better life in a land of greater opportunities. The settler migrant's ambition is not to return home wealthy, but to compete with his new peers and establish himself, and his children, in as much security as possible in the new country. From the viewpoint of the receiving country this motive is no more 'altruistic' than that of the *Gastarbeiter*, but there is a vast difference in willingness to assimilate. The decision to emigrate permanently is not taken lightly, and once taken it is invested with considerable emotional significance. The settler will want to prove that he made the right decision, and is therefore predisposed to be optimistic. His disillusionment with the 'old country' helps him to take a positive view of things that are new and different, and make conscious efforts to accommodate himself to them. He may over-identify, adopting new modes with incongruous enthusiasm, and be embarrassed by any of his compatriots who have not yet 'found their way around' and cling to old ways or make themselves conspicuous. His adaptation may be entirely successful, or it may be rather superficial, achieved only by denial and suppression of underlying emotion. If things do not work out as he had hoped, his reaction is likely to take the form of paranoid projection. It is not he who has failed, it is the country which has turned out to be different from what he was led to believe, or it is the natives who are prejudiced against him (true or not), or it was his wife who 'couldn't settle'. This should not surprise us, since by the act of emigration he gave an initial clue that he might be the kind of person who looks for the causes of his problems in his environment rather than within himself. It is not, however, necessary for the settler to repudiate his origins entirely. Once he has made the transition and re-established himself in the new country he can afford to be nostalgic again.

Settler migration is subject to stringent controls. Every country in the world reserves the right to screen potential settlers and select only those whose presence will benefit the country. In a world of autonomous nation-states this seems to be a legitimate function of national governments. The main receiving countries have traditionally been the United States, Canada, and Australia; with the post-war addition of Israel, these four received 73 per cent of international migration in the period 1918–54 (cited by Beijer, in Jackson 1969). In sharp contrast to *Gastarbeiters*, about half of settler-migrants are potential wage-earners (the others being wives and children) and of those, half are professionally qualified or skilled workers.

For economic reasons, post-war Britain has not attracted this type of settler in large numbers: the flow has been out rather than in. A good deal of the published literature on migrant adaptation comes from studies of settlers, and should not be applied unthinkingly to Britain.

Exiles

Refugees are a world phenomenon and a persistent one — a problem that has been described as a 'cumulative nightmare'. Twenty-five years after the end of the last war the UN estimated than over 45 million people had been forcibly displaced in that period — comparable to the total population of Britain. In 1979 the estimate of *current* refugees in the world was ten million. The social and psychological problems of refugees are considered in a separate chapter, but they differ from both *Gastarbeiters* and settlers in demography, motivation, the reception they receive on arrival, and their attitudes to long-term integration. Some become 'settlers' quite rapidly, others live only for the day when they can return. The post-war epidemiological studies, which showed refugees to have high rates of mental breakdown, have been applied unthinkingly to other categories of migrants, which is unwise.

Gastarbeiter or settler: conflict and ambiguity

In terms of motivation and attitude, the young man who came to Britain from (for example) Pakistan, fits the description of a *Gastarbeiter* as given above. He did not envisage remaining permanently in Britain: he left his family at home, and was prepared to put up with poor conditions and long hours of work in order to send money home. His aim was to accumulate wealth to improve the standing of his extended family at home. He took jobs that the English worker did not want (for example, in the textile mills on permanent night shifts), and he found cheap accommodation in a house belonging to a relative or fellow-villager who had preceded him. He was not motivated to learn English or understand English culture, or to modify his own behaviour any more than was necessary to avoid conflict. His emotional roots remained in Pakistan. But because he was given the legal status of a settler, he had the right to bring his wife and family to join him in Britain, and whenever this happens, other influences begin to be felt. Many of the original Indian and Pakistani immigrants still cherish the thought of returning 'home', and adopt an isolationist attitude to British society. They view much of British culture with misgiving, and are determined to hold on to their own traditions. Indeed, their nostalgia for the culture that they left frequently blinds them to the changes that have occurred in their absence; the culture they remember no longer exists. This creates the paradox that some aspects of Indian and Pakistani culture live on in Britain when India and Pakistan have altered: in some ways the expatriate community is more jealous of its traditions than the home community (a situation which could also be observed among expatriate Britons in outposts of empire). It is not difficult to understand this. Culture (as defined in Chapter 2) provides not only a blueprint for behaviour, but a meaning-system, a basis for moral judgments, and a sense of security — and these are never more precious to the individual than when he is adrift in an alien and confusing environment. Yet at the same time, he (and also, particularly, his children) is affected by British society. If he never learned English, his children do, and he cannot prevent them from being exposed to new ideas however uneasy that makes him. He finds that he is forced to make compromises and adaptations (Dahya 1973: Anwar 1979).

For many, this process takes place slowly by a series of adjustments and conflicts that are only part-recognized and part-resolved. Quite often an immigrant retains the *Gastarbeiter* mentality, the kinship loyalties, and the dream of return until he actually goes back for a visit. Then he realizes that his nostalgic dreams do not match reality, and that he himself has changed by being away, and he recognizes sadly that he and his family could not fit in 'back home'. After that he may acknowledge that England is now 'home', and start to make moves toward becoming a settler. Much the same process affects the refugee except that he is prevented from visiting 'home' to experience the change. There are Poles and Ukrainians who still regard themselves as exiles after thirty years; by contrast, the Ugandan Asians, who arrived having had a brutal lesson in what can happen to groups who maintain their own separateness in the face of a hostile majority, were anxious to become settlers as soon as possible, and took every opportunity to study English ways and adapt themselves to them.

Stoneqvist (1937) described the 'marginal man', who finds himself stranded between two cultures unable to identify fully with either, and this is a useful concept to apply in the field of immigration. Park (1928) had previously described the:

> 'sense of moral dichotomy and conflict [which] is probably char-
> acteristic of every immigrant during the period of transition, when
> old habits are being discarded and new ones are not yet formed. It is
> inevitably a period of inner turmoil and intensive self-consciousness.'
>
> (Park 1928 : 122)

The *Gastarbeiter* may not experience the feeling of marginality when he first arrives, but only when he starts the transition from self-image *Gastarbeiter* to self-image settler, which could be insidious and unrecognized, and many years later. The state of 'marginality' is a distressful one, and it is usually resolved by the adoption of one of the identity-options and abandonment of the other. This takes time and effort, and the conflicts that it creates lie at the roots of many of the problems that confront the practitioner. Those who say lightly, 'They have come here, they must conform to our ways', do not realize how laborious the task may be. The individual immigrant may not manage his transition from *Gastarbeiter* to settler on the basis of clear-thinking and logical decisions. Instead, he may muddle his way through with reluctant compromises and gnawing self-doubt – sometimes punctuated by inappropriate emotional outbursts.

In a way, the conflict faced by this individual is a paradigm for the conflicts of the whole society. Britain invited immigrants as a matter of economic expediency. To what extent are the indigenous British prepared to tolerate enclaves within society of citizens whose behaviour and allegiancies are unlike those of the majority? On the other hand, to what extent is it fair to expect a Pakistani or a Cypriot or a Ukrainian to turn his back on the cultural values of his upbringing and abandon traditions that support his emotional security? We, too, have tended to muddle our way through with reluctant compromises and gnawing self-doubt, punctuated by inappropriate emotional outbursts.

NOTES

1 These introductory descriptions are not comprehensive and are supplemented by specific references in later chapters. In addition to the authors cited, general background information may be found in Jackson (1969), Domnitz (1971), Nicolson (1974), Watson (1977), Holmes (1978), and Saifullah Khan (1979). Useful Bibliographies are those by Madan (1979), Runnymede Trust (n.d.).

4

Peasant Culture

Before proceeding to discuss specific adjustment problems it may be helpful to focus attention on those migrants to industrial countries who come from remote rural areas where the progress of education and economic development are slowest and the old traditions strongest. This applies especially to some who came as *Gastarbeiters* (even if they later became settlers). As well as the values specific to each culture, such people bring with them some attitudes that are common to rural communities, and which we may describe as *peasant attitudes*. Some of these attitudes are characteristic of closed communities in general.

The word 'peasant' is not intended to be pejorative or synonymous with 'primitive'. Peasant societies are complex and highly structured, with sophisticated value systems and formalized patterns of behaviour that make very good sense in their own context. The villager who migrates to the city, whether in his own country or overseas, has to adjust to the differences between rural and urban life. The original migrant is probably not a typical villager. He probably has unusual ambition and initiative, as well as access to sufficient material resources for the journey. This need not be true of his wife, brother, or other relative whom he sponsored to join him.

Not for one moment do we suggest that all immigrants in Britain are, or were, peasants. Some from Poland, Ukraine, India, Pakistan, and Bangla Desh may be so described, others not. In this chapter we are concerned with general statements, and it is interesting to learn that despite climatic and other differences, there are similarities between the peasant societies of India and Pakistan (Wiser and Wiser 1951; Carstairs 1958a; Bailey 1966; Saifullah Khan 1977, 1979; Carstairs and Kapur 1976), Spain (Aceves 1971), Italy (Friedman 1958), Poland (Thomas and Znaniecki 1918; Dobrowolski 1971), Algeria (Bordieu 1963), and Mexico (Lewis 1951; Foster 1965): and some of these common attributes were detectable quite recently in parts of Britain (Williams 1956; Hoggart 1958). The cultures of the Carribbean Islands are 'peasant' only in certain respects, because the background of slavery and the plantation economy had its own effects (Marshall 1968).

There are many definitions of the word peasant (Ortiz 1971). We are interested in the interactions of community members and their relationships with the world outside more than with patterns of land tenure so we can expand the term to include fishermen and other rural craftsmen. We shall define peasant societies as (among other things) rural primary producers which have some self-sufficiency, but have an economic relationship with a contiguous mercantile society on which they are in some ways dependent (Kroeber 1948; Foster 1973). This excludes, for example, tribesmen. Peasant societies are usually pre-literate, pre-scientific, and pre-industrial. They tend to rely 'exclusively on oral tradition and direct demonstration in handing down their cultural contents and experience' (Dobrowolski 1971 : 279).

All peasants are, in a sense, craftsmen. Rural manual work may be strenuous but it is not so repetitive and unthinking as most unskilled industrial work. In the course of a working day, a peasant performs many different tasks, each one involving some skill. Whether cutting sugar-cane, hauling in a fishing net, raking hay from a meadow, or milking a cow, there is a right way to do it — 'right' meaning efficient, garnering as much of the product as possible without squandering time or energy. The proper deployment of such skills is a source of pride and prestige (lost, of course, when the peasant becomes unskilled labour on the production line). Practical skills are learned by copying, not by theorizing. A young man who tries to find a new way to do some small task will find, more often than not, that at the end of the day he has accomplished less than his father, with more effort. A crop is planted at a particular time and in a particular way; there are certainly some reasons for doing so, based on trial and error in previous generations — but they are not known as 'reasons' and therefore cannot be discussed. There is no corpus of *theoretical* knowledge. The newcomer or innovator who asks, 'why?' will be told simply that it has always been so. The peasant is unwilling to deviate from tradition because he believes that his predecessors knew what they were about, and unless some new technology is available he is probably right. He senses that by introducing changes into part of the system he may upset some unseen equilibrium in the system as a whole, and in this, too, he is often right. Such equilibria may be defined in religious or superstitious terms, and because logical reasons are not available, the force of tradition itself acquires an inherent authority.

PEASANT CONFORMISM

'In peasant society conservatism appears generally to be culturally sanctioned.'

(Foster 1973 : 84)

In Poland:

'a tendency which is essentially conservative and stabilising . . . a propensity for the preservation of the existing social order. It is always based on the acknowledgement of previous experience and is essentially focussed on the past.'   (Dobrowski 1971 : 278)

'The permanent unchanging character of social institutions developed, implying belief in their intrinsic value. "Thus our fathers have done, thus we shall do", is a statement . . . which is often heard from peasants of the old traditional culture. In these circumstances any conscious rational motivation for economic activity or manner of conduct was of little relevance.'   (Dobrowolski 1971 : 287)

For the Algerian peasant:

'The future is not robbed of its menace unless it can be attached to and reduced to the past, until it can be lived as a simple continuation and accurate copy of the past . . . "If you resemble your father you cannot be accused of fault".'

(Bourdieu 1963, quoted in Foster 1973 : 84)

The group studied by Carstairs in Rajasthan would not regard themselves as peasants, but the same conformism is very clear:

'Acceptance of one's place in the caste system was unquestioning. It was a part of the order of nature. As a consequence of this, there was little room for ambition. . . . The old system puts a premium on conformity at the expense of personal initiative: the individual achieves integration and stability in his life habits by adhering to the pattern of his enveloping society, rather than by asserting his own personality.'   (Carstairs 1958a : 146)

In contemporary Britain it may be true that *asserting one's own personality* has been taken to extremes: we are experiencing 'future shock' (Toffler 1970) and are beginning to realize belatedly that 'Small is Beautiful' (Schumacher 1974). But even if the folk-wisdom is sometimes vindicated, when some apparently pointless ritual turns out to have a practical basis, or a scientific innovation has unforeseen side-effects, we must beware of taking too romantic a view. There are plenty of examples of traditional practices, sanctified by religious authority, that impede progress and perpetuate poverty, to the frustrated fury of those who work in development agencies. Peasant resistance to change is neither a virtue nor a vice, but merely a fact. The point is not whether the peasant dictum: 'Do what your father did, or you'll come to no good' is correct or not, but that in situations where survival is precarious, where there is no theory of cause and effect, and where advances are made by trial and error, such a dictum is inevitable. To carry on as we have always done is at least safe. To do differently might be better, but it might be worse, and if one is living at subsistence level that risk is too great.

THE CONTROL OF DEVIANCE

Conformism must be backed up by strong sanctions against deviance, and such sanctions will apply not only to food production but to other aspects of behaviour and social organization. The authority of elders is one controlling force. Ths is often remarked in Muslim culture, but it is a characteristic of peasant societies generally. Dobrowolski writes of: 'the patriarchal family and kinship which was expressed in the father's authority and power over children, in the children's economic and intellectual dependence upon parents, and the young people's submissive attitude' (Dobrowolski 1971 : 281). In British society it is permissible and indeed incumbent on young people to challenge tradition, oppose parental authority, and dismantle with glee any propositions that cannot withstand logical analysis. In peasant terms such behaviour is alarming, not merely because it jolts the confidence of the older generation, but because in some fundamental way, at a deeper level — which is quite valid in the context of peasant experience — it is socially destructive. The Muslim girl in Britain who challenges her parents' choice of husband is challenging the whole system of peasant thought, on which the group's emotional security is based; no wonder she is punished harshly.

Peer-group scrutiny and criticism is another means of social control: 'Concern with public opinion is one of the most striking characteristics of peasant communities' (Foster 1973). The myth of the close-knit rural community rich in mutual support and good fellowship does not stand up to inspection. Villages are as full of malice and coercion as any other community: 'Gossip is unrelenting and harsh . . . Facts about people are unconsciously or maliciously distorted . . . Relatives and neighbours are quick to believe the worst, and motives are always in question' (Lewis 1951 : 429); 'the Castillian peasant frequently views his world as a place where trouble lurks at every turn: a world of suspicions and mistrust, where order is a tenuous thing, difficult to achieve and more difficult to maintain' (Aceves 1971 : 127), quoted by Foster, who has collected similar statements from Mexico, Calabria, India, Peru, Slovenia, and China (Foster 1973 : 34).

Group pressure is perhaps a characteristic of all closed communities, especially those which are under siege from a harsh physical or social environment. Much the same thing was said about the Leeds working class in 1957: 'The group . . . imposes on its members an extensive and sometimes harsh pressure to conform . . . Working-class people watch and are watched in a manner which, because horizons are limited, will often result in a mistaken, and lowering, interpretation of what neighbours do' (Hoggart 1957 : 64). The intensity of neighbour-watching might have decreased a little, but malicious gossip and scandalmongering certainly live on, not only in the white population, but among the coloured newcomers who have joined them in the backstreets of Leeds.

An innovator may be rejected and punished even when his innovation is successful — perhaps especially if it is successful: 'successful persons are popular targets of criticism, envy, and malicious gossip' (Lewis 1951, on Mexican peasants). Bailey states bluntly that in his Indian village:

'success — spectacular success — is attributed to human wickedness. The man, who, as we say, makes a killing, is not reaping the rewards of hard work and correct calculation, but made his way through sorcery and magic or at least in some way which was harmful to his fellows. Judging by the stories I was told of how men in Bisipara first became wealthy, the peasant mythology contains no category of honest riches . . . any peasant who becomes rich must have cheated, must have exploited his fellow, and to that extent should be punished or put outside the moral community.'

(Bailey 1966 : 314)

'THE IMAGE OF LIMITED GOOD'

This cynicism is accounted for by Foster in his concept of 'the image of limited good' (Foster 1967). According to this, peasant attitudes to all goods are conditioned by their attitude to the basic resource, which is land. Since in any community the amount of cultivable land is limited — or at least the peasant can see no way of increasing it — he is predisposed to regard all resources as limited: not to be increased, but only to be divided in different ways. It follows that if one member of the community is seen to be doing well, acquiring wealth, this must be at the expense of others. If it is not obvious how the trick is done, witchcraft is the usual explanation.

The mentality of mutual distrust which is characteristic of peasant societies is vividly exemplified by the Wisers' description:

'We fear the rent collector, we fear the police watchman, we fear everyone who looks as if he might claim some authority over us, we fear our creditors, we fear our patrons, we fear too much rain, we fear locusts, we fear thieves, we fear the evil spirits which threaten our children and our animals, and we fear the strength of our neighbours.   (Wiser and Wiser 1951 : 160)

The general rule is: do not allow yourself to fall behind the average standards of the group, as this will be an invitation to exploitation, *but* do not appear to be getting ahead either because success indicates malpractice. Success, moreover, carries the risk of actual attack. It is prudent to conceal wealth. Speaking of the mud walls of India, the Wisers say:

'our fathers built them strong . . . but they are a better protection if instead of being strong they are allowed to become dilapidated. Dilapidation makes it harder for the covetous visitor to tell who is actually poor and who simulates poverty. When men become strong, they . . . dare to expose their prosperity in walls of better materials and workmanship. But if the ordinary man suddenly makes his wall conspicuous, the extortioner is on his trail . . . old walls tell no tales.'
(Wiser and Wiser 1951 : 157, quoted by Foster 1973 : 37)

It may be that the penalizing of success in peasant society provides a stimulus to emigration by the more imaginative, innovative, or impatient members. There is, of course, no restriction on making money out of strangers! Perhaps we can discern here one of the origins of that entrepreneurial flair which seems to be displayed so often by migrants. There is a bonus back home, because remittances sent home by the emigre worker are 'windfalls'. They come from outside the community, so they are exempt from the restrictions of 'limited good', and can be utilized to advance the position of a family without provoking too much resentment. (But some sharing is expected, and the giving of presents or feasts may be acts of propitiation and symbolic or actual redistribution.)

Material wealth is a 'limited good', but so are other kinds of good fortune. The man who is blessed with strong sons, or good health, provokes envy; and not only envy but suspicion that somehow or other he has contrived to gain these blessings at someone else's expense. By the same token, anyone who is failing to prosper or suffers illness or infertility, easily attributes these misfortunes to witchcraft.

LEADERSHIP

Reluctance to step out of line may stifle initiative in other ways too. The peasant is unwilling to be a leader or organizer:

> 'He feels — for good reason — that his motives will be suspect and that he will be subject to the criticism of neighbours. By seeking, or even accepting, an authority position, the ideal man ceases to be ideal. A "good" man therefore usually shuns community responsibilities (other than of a ritual nature): by so doing he protects his reputation.'   (Foster 1967 : 313)

Plainly, this is too sweeping a statement to be universal: there are co-operative self-help schemes in operation with acknowledged leadership to offset the many sad accounts of community development failures.

Among immigrant groups in Britain there are those who might be expected to take a lead in a community who conspicuously decline to do so, but on the other hand there are others who are very willing to adopt leadership roles in public (sometimes without ensuring that they have any followers). A member of an ethnic minority who is placed — or places himself — in a position of public prominence, has many other pressures on him and is probably a person who has moved a long way from his peasant background, if he ever had one. However, an ambivalent attitude *to* him by others in the group might have something to do with peasant attitudes.

ATTITUDES TO TIME

Another characteristic commonly described in peasant cultures is their attitude to time. In the short term, punctuality and strict obedience to the clock are less important in non-industrial societies. Work stops when the task is completed; buses depart when they are full; people who do not carry engagement diaries are less put out if they have to wait for an hour and more willing to put aside what they were doing to entertain a visitor or help a friend. In the longer term there is, according to some writers, a different attitude to the future, and therefore to the making of plans.

Bordieu (1963) distinguishes what he calls 'the round of time' which is a peasant concept, from 'the arrow of time' which urban man uses for planning. To a peasant, things come in cycles: daylight defines the working day (artificial lighting at night is expensive); seasons recur predictably; and there are longer cycles too — so many years before the ox must be replaced, or the thatch, so many years before the son

replaces the father, and so on. The expectation is that after an appropriate interval, situations will come round again much as they are now,
and planning is on this basis. Major changes, sequential, directional —
what we call development — are not expected.

Urban man has a different attitude:

'Those who make five-year plans are thinking of time as an arrow.
The work has a beginning and an end: there is a target to be reached.
The end is a state of affairs quite different from the beginning, and
is itself a starting point for further ventures. We have no difficulties
with this notion. To plan a future state of affairs which is radically
different from the present is to us quite rational. But those who
think in terms of the round of time see such changes as coming from
mystical forces like fate, or luck, or witchcraft or acts of God, and
to plan for such events makes nonsense. The politician who promises
a good life in store for everyone if they help to implement the plan,
is heard by the peasants as we would hear a man promising everyone
a first dividend on the pools every week.'

(Bailey 1971 — 315–16)

This distinction between 'cyclic' and 'developmental' changes is related
to the extent to which people feel themselves to be in control of their
own futures. In one study, questions about the future were put to
farmers whose land was not irrigated (and therefore dependent on
variations in rainfall), and to farmers who had irrigated land. Those who
had the relative security of irrigation had plans for the future: those
without replied: 'What God wills' (Myren, cited in Ortiz 1971).

ATTITUDE TO OUTSIDERS

We may think that in their dealings with each other, peasants appear
somewhat paranoid: it is a cultural paranoia, important to the psychiatrist only because he must make allowances for it. But if they view each
other with suspicion, this is nothing to the way they view outsiders: 'It
is not permissible to beat the people from our own village, but the
people from other villages can, and should, be beaten' (Dobrowolski
1971 : 294).

Polish emigrants in the early years of the century tended to stay
together, village by village, in the cities of America. They found work if
possible in the same factories (Thomas and Znaniecki 1918). In precisely
the same way, post-war migrants to Britain tended to settle in certain
cities; and not only Mirpuris in Bradford and Bengalis in East London,
but, if possible, people from the same village in the same area of the
city. Many co-villagers are also relatives, but even those who are not

related cluster together and are sometimes referred to in Britain as brother, or 'village brother'. West Indians arriving in London would usually seek out someone from the same island (Selvon 1956) and even twenty years later there are communities of Barbadians, Kittitians, Montserratians, and so on, who take care to keep in touch with each other:

> 'Consequently, not only do Montserratians tend to live in certain urban neighbourhoods but kin and friends from the same parts of the island often cluster in the same houses and streets within those areas. For example, migrants from a village in eastern Montserrat who are mostly settled in Stoke Newington, often refer to Birmingham as "Long Ground" because that is where most of the migrants from a nearby village of that name in Montserrat live.'
>
> (Philpott 1977 : 108)

Turkish *Gastarbeiters* in Germany follow the same pattern, with particular employers drawing from individual villages (Berger and Mohr 1975). In a Bradford textile mill, employment vacancies are often filled by an existing employee who introduces a 'village brother': and the personnel manager accepts this because he has found that such groups work well together, whereas if he insists on introducing an 'outsider' problems may arise and the outsider often leaves.

The insularity and exclusiveness of closed communities is not confined to peasants. Williams found it in the North of England in 1956:

> 'The people of Gosforth make a sharp distinction between "Gosfer folk" and those who live outside the parish . . . very apparent in attitudes towards "offcomers" . . . More often than not the new family's first few months in the parish are marked by a combination of hospitality and hostility, of co-operation and criticism . . . the apparent ambivalence . . . is very puzzling to newcomers, many of whom describe it in such terms as "stabbing you in the back" or "being two-faced".'

> '. . . two farmers . . . came to the parish at about the same time. The first, is a second cousin to two local farmers and more distantly related to several other people in the parish. Although not personally known to the majority of people this farmer appears to have been accepted very rapidly indeed, and the process of settling in seems to have taken place with very little criticism and hostility. The second farmer was born in the south of England, had never farmed before he came to Gosforth, and was not related or known to anyone in the parish. He speaks with what is locally termed a "la-ti-posh" accent and retains a great many of the urban habits and values he acquired

before coming to Cumberland. After nearly seven years this farmer has clearly not "settled down". He is the subject of slanderous stories by a large number of people and is still in many ways as much an offcomer as on the day he came.' (Williams 1956 : 168-70)

ATTITUDE TO EXTERNAL AUTHORITIES

Peasants reserve their greatest paranoia for outsiders who represent authority. Their belief is that external authority, by and large, does not mean well by them. An extreme example of this is given by Curle:

'A Pakistani friend of mine, a wise and humane administrator, was driving through a village when a little girl ran suddenly in front of his car. He rushed the badly hurt child to the nearest hospital, but she died on the way, and he took her back, grieving. He fully expected to be mobbed by the angry villagers, but was so distressed that he did not mind. However, the girl's grandfather simply said, "God has taken our child; that cannot be undone. We ask nothing of you except that you should not tell the police. If you do they will come here to make an investigation. They will stay for weeks; they will eat all our chickens. They will find out all about us and blackmail us: if anyone protests, he will be beaten and taken to jail.'
(Curle 1971 : 87)

There are immigrant groups in Britain who view the British police with as much misgiving, not because they are peasants (most of them are not), but for immediate and important reasons to be considered later. The culture of a closed community, however, adds to this. Even among Cumberland farmers, who had less reason to feel threatened by authority, Williams found a paranoid response (which in this case has its amusing side):

'Much of the hostility and suspicion I encountered in the early stages of the field work were due to the fact that I was believed to be variously an Inspector of the Ministry of Agriculture, an official of the Inland Revenue, a Rates Assessor for the Rural District Council, or simply an unspecified "bloody Nosey Parker from some office". Instances of the way these officials are treated are plentiful. Several people told me of the farmer who took a representative of "Ministry" up on horseback to a very remote fell pasture to see some of his animals, and then returned alone, leaving the unfortunate man to walk back. This was locally regarded as very amusing and its telling was normally garnished with such remarks as "Ah doubt he nivver learned about that at college".'

'In all such stories the local inhabitant outwits the visiting official and the greater the discomfiture of the latter, the better the story.'
(Williams 1956 : 170)

In this case the hostility to officialdom was not a matter of social classs — Gosforth farmers were by no means poverty-stricken or oppressed — but it can also be a class issue. Hoggart noted:

'a common attitude which causes working-class people only to make use of "Them" when absolutely forced: if things go wrong . . . put up with them: don't get into the hands of authority, and if you must have help, only "trust your own sort".

'It starts from the feeling that life is hard and that "our sort" will usually get "the dirty end of the stick".'   (Hoggart 1958 : 56)

Typical peasant strategy is not to confront authority, but to circumvent it. Peasants do not shout their grievances or demand their rights: they discover ways of succeeding in spite of the rules. They hope that the official will go away soon and leave them alone, and in the meantime the rule is: *tell him as little as possible.* The less 'they' know about you, the less harm they can do you. Information is a valuable commodity, not to be squandered. Williams's Gosforth study coincided with a national census, and he noted people's reluctance to fill in their census forms:

'Many regard it as quite pointless and quite a number as a devious method of obtaining information for tax purposes . . . not a few of the returns were deliberately falsified "to give 'em summat to puzzle on". My attempts at explaining the uses of the Census were often regarded with open disbelief or dismissal in such terms as "Well, it's time they found something more useful to spend their money on I fancy". It was quite clear that a large number of people looked on the Census as an unwarranted intrusion into their affairs, and in some vague and unforeseeable way as a threat to the wellbeing of the individual and the community. As one housewife remarked: "I still can't see why them London folk wants to know ivverything about ivverybody in Gosfer".'   (Williams 1956 : 173)

If the writers of spy stories are to be believed, the secret services function on a 'need to know' basis. Peasants have always functioned on that basis. Information is a 'limited good'. The peasant's defence against authority is a blank stare.[2]

PEASANT ATTITUDES AND THE PRACTITIONER

The implications of this for the practitioner are obvious. The doctor or social worker who tries conscientiously to obtain a detailed social history, and attempts to record the names, ages, and other details of every member of the family is pretty certain to meet a blank look. The patient has forgotten, or suddenly ceases to understand English. Polite small-talk with enquiries about absent relatives or conditions back home may be regarded as snooping. Anyone whose role is not clearly defined and recognized – such as a health visitor or school liaison officer – may be a spy for the police, or Home Office immigration department, or 'them'. Even the doctor, whose role is accepted, arouses suspicion if he takes too much interest in illnesses of the past, which, in the patient's view, have no relevance to the present.

Again, there is a social class element to this: 'working-class people often seem not "oncoming" to social workers, seem evasive and prepared to give answers designed to put off rather than to clarify' (Hoggart 1958 : 59). Hoggart interpreted this as hurt pride, reluctance to disclose shameful need. It is as likely to be a simple reflex reaction. The uninitiated enquirer notices the hesitancy and defensiveness, and assumes that the client is hiding something: and may embark on fantasies about social security frauds or illegal immigrants or all manner of deceptions – or simply decide that the respondent is sly and untrustworthy. Thus, paranoia begets paranoia, and communication comes to an end.

Some of the unflattering stereotypes that white society projects on to immigrants are that they are exclusive; stay with their own kind; don't join in things; stick to their old ways; don't tell you what they really think; are secretive or downright deceitful; parsimonious; grasping; crafty; unreliable. If there is truth in these criticisms, the attributes probably have more to do with the fact that they are peasants than with being Pakistani, or black, or whatever. Industrial societies find it convenient to import cheap labour to do unskilled jobs. To import cheap labour is very often to import peasants, and it is only to be expected that peasants will have peasant characteristics.

At the same time, some immigrants – especially Asians – are derided because they have not stood up for their rights, have not protested against discrimination and victimization, have stayed in the shadows and walked close to the wall instead of coming out to fight against the system; but those are also peasant strategies, and should not surprise us. They are beginning to alter, and their children especially are learning fast how to complain, demonstrate, and confront.

NOTES

1 Therefore in recording a client's background the practitioner should always ask: City? Town? Village? There may be some reluctance to admit a village background. The response 'Lahore', 'Rawalpindi', etc., is not specific: it may refer to the city or the rural district (Tehsil) of that name. Jamaicans prefer to claim that they came from Kingston, rather than from a village.

2 Well portrayed in the painting 'Le Petit Paysan'. Modigliani 1917 (Tate Gallery).

Adjustment

5

Dislocation

Human beings appreciate a sense of *belonging*. We value our roots in a *place* with familiar landmarks and personal associations, and in a *group* with people whose behaviour we understand and with whom we need not be on guard. To belong is not merely comforting, but an important ingredient of personal identity. The familiar environment reassures me that I am the person I think I am. *Integration* into a group, and the *integrity* of the self, are linked concepts. In one ancient language, the noun for 'home' is the same word as the verb 'I am'.[1]

Therefore uprooting, especially separation from both place and group at the same time, is an inherently stressful business. Migration is an adventure in which excitement may play a part, but so do anxiety and a sense of loss, and sometimes the latter predominate. The stresses are greatest if the journey is long and complicated (making 'escape' more difficult), it is undertaken alone, and there are large differences in culture and problems of language to contend with. A young girl born in Kashmir may have never left her village before she sets out for Britain, nor crossed a busy street until she arrives in Rawalpindi. She may never have seen an aeroplane until she gets on one, and never seen so many people all together in one place as she will encounter at London Airport. This description fits only a small minority of the immigrants who have arrived in recent years, but it does fit a few of them, even now. It is not surprising if they arrive bewildered, perplexed and distressed. A refugee may arrive exhausted and confused, having lived with extreme fear for the preceding weeks or months, his mind filled with kaleidoscopic memories of destruction and horror. Even the most robust and self-possessed person is unlikely to have complete command of his or her emotions at such a time. Psychological defence mechanisms take over: irrational behaviour may take the observer and the subject himself by surprise; feelings of fear, or love, hatred, anger, or dependency may become displaced on to inappropriate recipients; trivial incidents become magnified into major issues; slight setbacks and misunderstandings seem like disasters. Some defend themselves against their own anxiety by retreating into a world of fantasy or nostalgia, or even into a condition of partial dissociation such that they move through the whole experience 'like zombies' and have only hazy recollections afterwards. Others remain in a condition of heightened arousal with sharpened perceptions, and can recall the whole experience in tremendous detail.

These are just some of the possible reactions at and soon after arrival. They are not difficult to imagine or understand (though it must be said that if immigration officials at the ports of arrival in Britain possess such imagination and understanding, most of them succeed in concealing it). What is less obvious — but becomes apparent later — is that even when the immediate stages of adaptation have been completed successfully, and the subject appears to be comfortably settled into his new environment, the old feelings of loss, or despair, or homesickness, or anger, can be *reactivated* by a new stimulus. Such a stimulus might be related — for example a letter or visitor from home, especially if the news from home is worrying — or unrelated, such as having to go into hospital to have a baby. At such a time, even years after the event, the old conflicting emotions may come back to the surface and produce changes of mood or incongruous behaviour.

'CULTURE SHOCK'

The term 'culture shock' was first popularized by Oberg (1954) and has been used to describe some of the problems of American Peace Corps Volunteers and technologists living in 'Third World' countries (Foster 1973). The concept is applicable in part to travel in the opposite direction. Culture shock happens when the psychological cues that help an individual to function in society are withdrawn and replaced by new ones. These cues include:

'the thousand and one ways in which we orient ourselves to the situations of daily life: when to shake hands and what to say when we meet people, when and how to give tips, how to give orders . . . how to make purchases . . . when to take statements seriously and when not. Now these cues which may be words, gestures, facial expressions, customs, or norms are acquired by all of us in the course of growing up and are as much a part of our culture as the language we speak or the beliefs we accept. All of us depend for our peace of mind and our efficiency on hundreds of these cues, most of which we do not carry on the level of conscious awareness.'

(Oberg 1954, quoted in Foster 1973 : 192)

Oberg and Foster both refer to culture shock as a malady, a kind of 'mental illness' which is an occupational 'disease' of living abroad. The symptoms (in the case of the Peace Corps Volunteer) are said to include excessive preoccupation with the purity of food and drink, fear of physical contact with natives, great concern with minor pains and skin eruptions, excessive anger over trivial frustrations, a paranoid belief that one is being cheated, feelings of helplessness and inadequacy combined with refusal to learn the local language, desire for the company of ones own 'kind', and:

> 'that terrible longing to be back home, to be able to have a good cup of coffee and a piece of apple pie, to walk into that corner drugstore, to visit one's relatives, and in general, to talk to people who really make sense.'   (Oberg 1954 : 2–3, cited by Foster 1973 : 191)

We might quibble about describing these reactions as a 'disease', since they are said to be, in some measure, universal. Obviously the symptoms will vary according to the situation (for coffee and apple pie, read fresh mangoes or sea eggs), but the general point is valid. According to Foster, culture shock cannot be entirely avoided by being broad-minded and full of goodwill. These attributes 'may aid in recovery, but they can no more prevent the illness than grim determination can prevent a cold' (Foster 1973 : 192). Foster identifies various stages of the 'disease':

> 'During the first, or incubation stage, the victim may feel positively euphoric . . . it is clear that a wonderful experience lies ahead. The new arrival notices colleagues who have been on duty a few months who seem grouchy and depressed and ill-adjusted, and he may feel condescending about these poor fellows who have not yet made the adjustment that he, the new arrival, has accomplished all in a few days . . . Then. wham! The Cook's tour is over, and the virus bites deep. There is maid trouble, school trouble, language trouble, house trouble, transportation trouble, shopping trouble — trouble everywhere. All the things about everyday living which were taken for granted at home now become insurmountable problems . . . At this stage the victim bands together with his fellow sufferers to exchange symptoms and to criticise the host country and all its citizens . . . "These people can't plan", "They have no manners", "They ought to be taught how to get things done".'
>
>   (Foster 1973 : 192–93)

(Perhaps in Britain we might substitute: 'The British are all callous and stand-offish . . . they all hate foreigners . . . there is universal racial prejudice and discrimination . . . decadence . . . immorality . . . hypocrisy . . .')

The third, or recovery stage, begins when the newcomer begins to pick up some of the cues which orientate him, and at the same time some of the language.

> 'Little by little the problems of living are worked out and it becomes apparent that the situation, although difficult, is not as hopeless as it seemed a short time earlier. A returning sense of humour is helpful at this point; when the patient can joke about his sad plight, he is well on the road to recovery. . . . (Eventually) he comes to accept the customs of the country for what they are. He doesn't necessarily wax enthusiastic about all of them, but he doesn't chafe . . . The environment remains the same, but the technician adapts himself to it; it is his changed attitude that has restored his health.
>
> (Foster 1973 : 193–94)

In the situation described by these authors, the American volunteer has been 'thrown in at the deep end' and is more or less on his own. He is also an 'expert' and therefore in a privileged position. Neither of these two conditions apply to most immigrants to Britain. Most are in close contact with members of their own ethnic group. Knowledge of culture shock helps us to understand the importance of cultural support and the durability of ethnic enclaves.

An Asian, Cypriot, Vietnamese, or other minority family in Britain can protect itself against culture shock to some extent by avoiding contact with the world outside the ethnic enclave, by carrying on a traditional life as if one were still back home. (As did many a British family living in India.) But this cannot go on indefinitely. Sooner or later every immigrant has to emerge from sanctuary and make contact with the host society, be it at work, or school, or when there is illness or some problem that requires help from a statutory authority. It is possible for an immigrant (especially a woman who does not go out to work) to remain insulated for years, and then experience the full force of culture shock when the family moves from an inner-city enclave to a suburban housing estate; or when she goes into hospital to have a baby. Foster states that the 'disease' usually runs its course in a matter of months: 'Resilient people are over it in three months, not infrequently it goes on for a year. Few people, when experiencing it for the first time, are well recovered in less than six months' (Foster 1973 : 195). In Britain, it usually runs a less definite course, and 'relapses' may occur at any time.

LOSS OF ROLE IDENTITY

As well as deriving a sense of identity from a familiar environment and social group, most people gain reassurance from the enactment of familiar roles. Thus the surgeon who can carry out operations, or the mother who can feed her baby, feel more at ease in an alien environment than a person who has to start learning something completely new. To ply one's own trade, or deploy one's own personal skills, is not merely ego-boosting in a trivial sense, but also more fundamentally, since these are some of the criteria by which the self is distinguished from others, and personal identity reaffirmed. Every peasant is in some sense a craftsman (see Chapter 4): in Britain he becomes unskilled labour, probably carrying out some simple repetitive procedure which can be learned in half an hour and as quickly forgotten, and which anyone else could do just as well as he does. A more highly qualified immigrant (and there are many who have professional or technical qualifications) may well find that his talents are not required or his credentials not recognized, so he, too, is forced into the ranks of the unskilled, where he does not belong. Language alone may be a barrier to obtaining employment consistent with experience and previous status.

These factors of role-loss and status-loss bear particularly hard on adult men. Children and elderly people escape them, and so to some extent do women if they have a continuing role as wife, mother, or grandmother. There is some evidence that downward social mobility, in employment-status terms, is a factor in the incidence of mental illness among immigrant groups.

However, role-identity is not limited to employment. In an Indian family the elders have patriarchal (and in some respects matriarchal) authority. The head of the household enacts a particular role which will descend on his death to his eldest son. He has responsibility for arranging marriages, apportioning land or other family property, approving the plans and ambitions of children and grandchildren, and applying corrective discipline to any youngster who steps out of line and places the family honour in jeopardy. People come to him for advice, and value his wisdom. But in Britain such a man may discover that his wisdom is scorned, his judgement disregarded. His daughter or grand-daughter objects to his marriage plans; his son manages his affairs with the aid of solicitors and accountants; when domestic discords erupt into violence, a social worker appears on the scene. His social role is eroded. Similarly, a West Indian matron offers support to her young daughter or grand-daughter, or niece who has just had a baby. The old lady puts herself out to help the young mother, and to teach her from her own store of knowledge and experience. But here comes a health visitor with different ideas — and the old lady is disregarded.

Loss of meaningful roles is one of the components of the syndrome of *institutionalization* — the iatrogenic disorder that caused so many of the residents of the old-style mental hospital to sit all day sunk in apathy and inertia. 'What am I for?', if unanswered, leads easily to 'What am I?'.

THE NEED TO SUCCEED

All migrants travel in order to improve their lot. Students come to acquire an education, refugees to seek safety, most others to acquire wealth. Settlers are seeking a better life in the new country, migrant workers hope to have a better life on their return home. One way or another, *improvement* is the motive behind the upheaval. Great sacrifices have been made to achieve it, and if success is not forthcoming those sacrifices were in vain. The sacrifices include not only the loneliness, homesickness, culture-shock, role-change, and general insecurity, but also the actual expenditure of large sums of hard-saved cash. The young man who sets out boldly to seek his fortune in the gold-paved cities of Britain carries a heavy burden of responsibility and indebtedness – often an actual financial debt. To justify himself and repay his debt he *must* succeed – in actual financial terms.

Inevitably, many immigrants in all walks of life find that success eludes them. Promised jobs do not materialize; competition is greater than they could imagine; when work is available wages are certainly higher than back home, but the cost of living is very much higher still. Yet somehow money must be saved and sent back home in regular remittances to the family. Many a *Gastarbeiter* lives in severe poverty, but pride obliges him to maintain the pretence of success – he cannot tell his relatives that he is a failure. When he goes home for a visit he must take expensive presents for all the family, and display his wealth by his clothes, possessions, and behaviour. This kind of pretence imposes its own strains, increases the sense of isolation, prevents rational and detached appraisal of the situation, and perhaps encourages alienation from both worlds.

Similar problems often afflict the overseas student, whose aspirations may be unrealistic, but who simply *cannot* contemplate going home without the qualification he came to obtain. The refugee, whose need to reconstruct a life for himself has a different origin, usually requires material success as a part of that reconstruction.

LANGUAGE

Among the stresses that beset an immigrant, problems of communication merit particular mention and can hardly be overestimated. A person who is unable to understand what his neighbour is saying is more likely to become suspicious about the neighbour. He is at a disadvantage in everyday transactions, and dependent on the services of interpreters. It becomes extremely difficult to make new friends, or come to terms with the new culture. Some of the practical problems that complicate practitioner–client understanding (especially in psychiatry) are considered in later chapters. But linguistic isolation goes deeper than that. In its effects on the personality of the individual it has something in common with deafness, driving the sufferer in on himself, encouraging a self-centred and possibly idiosyncratic view of reality in which fantasies are not checked out and misunderstandings multiply. At the same time there is heightened sensitivity to non-verbal perceptions and the nuances of other people's behaviour, often misinterpreted. If communication is difficult, the habit of sharing thoughts and ideas may be lost, and with it the ability to make relationships. Deaf people not infrequently become paranoid, and so do people who are socially and linguistically isolated. Some more subtle consequences of linguistic deprivation have been described very clearly in the personal account of a British psychologist working in Denmark (Moore 1977).

NOTE

1   Cornish *bos* (n) home, (v) I am. The same root is detectable in Welsh.

Rejection

There is abundant evidence that ethnic minorities in Britain are at a disadvantage in every important socio-economic variable (Smith 1977; Community Relations Council 1977; Cross 1978; Scarman 1981; and many others). They experience prejudice and rejection in everyday situations, and the Race Relations Act devised for their protection touches only the tip of the iceberg. Insult is added to injury when they are accused of having caused the problems under which they suffer. Many settled in inner-city areas because housing was cheap, large Victorian houses suited extended-family lifestyles, and in any case they were barred from 'white' suburbia. Now they are accused of causing the decay of those areas — which were actually dilapidated before they arrived. They attend the most ill-equipped schools — and are then derided for failing in academic attainment. They are refused jobs — and then criticized for living on social security. Most of the criticisms are quite unfair. It is not the immigrants who have caused the defects in British society, it is truer to say that they act as a marker, identifying and rendering visible some of the defects that were already present in the structure.

Some who write and speak on behalf of ethnic minorities claim that victimization and exploitation are the causes of all their problems. These are (they say) the only issues worth discussing — and they are issues which practitioners systematically ignore.

> 'Black people are continuously under real stress because of the racism they encounter in their everyday lives — racial attacks for which police protection is not available, harrassment of black people on the streets by the police themselves, homes being invaded by the police who claim to be "looking for drugs" and passport raids . . . involving 50 police and immigration officers with dogs. This kind of stress caused strictly by the state was never mentioned by the

doctors we spoke to, instead they redefine it as "neurosis", an individual problem and, by implication, the individual's fault . . . in everything which has been written about "ethnic minorities" and health there is the same constant refrain: Black culture is to blame for people's ill health . . . all the "ethnic minorities" experts are saying the same thing: to improve black people's health their culture must be modified. This approach is not only racist, in that it assumes the superiority of their own white indigenous culture, it also actively obscures the social and economic roots of ill health among black people.'   (Wilson 1981)

This argument has considerable force. We must never underestimate the extent of the injustice suffered by minority groups, nor the sheer grinding unpleasantness of a life of rejection. But to say that all problems are due to racism, and nothing else should be discussed, seems somewhat of an oversimplification. 'Racism' has become a slogan word, more often shouted than analysed.

It may be true that Britain is a racist society, but before we accept that completely we should at least ask what the accusation means. Sociological and political factors are of crucial importance, but so are the psychological factors which underlie them. In terms of attitudes, racism is a composite that includes (among other things) *xenophobia, superiority, exclusiveness, authoritarianism,* and *prejudice.*

XENOPHOBIA

The British have always disliked foreigners. A post-war Polish refugee stated after ten years in Britain: 'the atmosphere of this country is such that it favours the formation of foreign ghettoes . . . in no country is the word foreigner so offensively pronounced' (Zubkzucki 1956). Jewish refugees at the turn of the century were described as 'rubbish'; 'smouldering fire . . . eating at the very vitals of the metropolis'; 'the scum washed to our shores in the dirty water flowing from foreign drainpipes'; and 'those loathsome wretches who come grunting and itching to our shores' (Nicolson 1974 : 100–01). Until this century Britain had always prided itself an offering refuge to the victims of oppression in less enlightened lands: but too many at a time, threatening to change the face of society even slightly, went beyond the limits of tolerance. It seemed outrageous that 'There are some streets you may go through and hardly know you are in England' (Nicolson 1974). So it has continued: every group of immigrants entering Britain this century has been subjected to public abuse sooner or later and even refugees whose publicized sufferings *en route* ensure them sympathy on arrival, find that the welcome is temporary. Scurrilous tales are told, and a mythology of vilification develops. In the 1880s it was asserted that synagogues were being built in prisons because there were so many Jewish criminals inside; in the 1980s leprosy was said to be endemic among Asian and West Indian immigrants (neither statement having any foundation).

Hostility is not confined to any sector of the community or political party. Ben Tillett said to the Jews 'You are our brothers, and we will do our duty by you. But we wish you had not come' (Nicolson 1974 : 101), and Trades Union attitudes have not altered much since then. Whatever the reasons, the British do not take a delight in cosmopolitanism.

SUPERIORITY

Among traditionalist Britons the belief dies hard that the British way of doing things is naturally the best. Though few would state it explicitly, it underlies many unconscious assumptions. The more 'tolerant' or 'liberal-minded' may concede that particular foreigners are rather better at a few specific things, but these are exceptions counterbalanced by many inferiorities. The ludicrous arrogance of this attitude has obvious historical roots, and it is particularly relevant to white-black relationships, as mentioned in various other chapters. Colonial administration justifies itself, like any other totalitarian regime, by the belief that the masses ('the natives') are incapable of governing themselves. By keeping them in an inferior position one can then deride them for being inferior, which justifies their continued subjugation.

EXCLUSIVENESS

Americans, when faced with massive immigration from Europe two generations ago, adopted a deliberate 'melting-pot' policy whereby every child learned at school what to do to become a Good American Citizen. The British have never offered this kind of induction. At one level this may be because we lack any clear sense of what a Good British Citizen would be (see below); but perhaps it also reflects a clique mentality. A clique is an exclusive group which takes pleasure in remaining exclusive. Mannerisms of speech, dress, and habits are used as social signals within the clique and barriers against those who aspire to join. People who are not admitted are never told why they are

unacceptable — in fact they are never told outright that they *are*
unacceptable⁻ — they are simply rejected or ignored. Clique-divisions
are often but not always coterminous with class-divisions and power-
hierarchies, and they are very subtle. The outsider is in a Catch-22
position: he cannot join without knowing the password, and no-one
will tell him the password or even admit that it exists.

AUTHORITARIANISM

In the social psychology of racism a seminal work is *The Authoritarian
Personality* (Adorno *et al.* 1950). A group of American workers set out
to discover what kind of people were racially prejudiced, what other
characteristics such people had, and whether their attitudes could be
understood as part of a more general analysis of personality. Their
research was concerned primarily with anti-semitism but the findings
have wider application.[1] In brief, they identified a personality-type
with the following salient characteristics:

(1) Conventionality: adherence to the conventional values of their
    society, a submissive attitude towards the moral authority of the
    society, and a tendency to look out for and condemn anyone who
    violates those conventions.
(2) Condemnation in particular of sexual deviation in any form.
(3) Preoccupation with power: a tendency to see all relationships in
    terms of strong-weak, dominance-submission parameters, and to
    extol the virtues of toughness and assertiveness and admire those
    attributes in leaders.
(4) Cynicism and pessimism about 'human nature': readiness to believe
    that society is controlled by conspiracies, and that wicked things
    are done in secret places.
(5) Rejection of reflective, contemplative, and aesthetic values, espec-
    ially innovative creativity.

The methodology of the original research is open to criticism (Brown
1965) but the general point is valid: these traits do tend to go together,
and they tend to go with a racist outlook though not all racists are
authoritarian (Wellman 1977). In extreme form, the profile of the
authoritarian personality fits very well the typical member of the
National Front if we can judge this from the statements made by its
spokesmen and in the pages of *Spearhead* in the days before such
statements were rendered illegal by the Race Relations Act. The
National Front and similar organizations are not merely anti-black
groups. They proclaim the moral virtues of a traditional society in

which the purity of an elite race was not contaminated by alien influences. They perceive an enormous conspiracy in which Jews, liberals, communists, international financiers, artists, intellectuals, and sexual perverts have seized control of the media and the universities and are hell-bent on destroying the moral values of 'ordinary decent people'. Their ideal society would be tough and puritanical, with emphasis on discipline, capital punishment, and a hard line with crime in general, an end to permissiveness, Welfare State largesse, pop culture, and birth control (Harris 1973). Such values are not peculiar to the National Front, nor is the world divided into authoritarian and anti-authoritarian factions. There is a continuum, and to a lesser degree we can detect authoritarianism in the public statements of many who repudiate Fascism as such. The continuum does not coincide with the left-right continuum of politics – there is an authoritarianism of the extreme left as well as the extreme right – nor is it dependent on social class or level of education. Anyone can probably recognize members of their own circle, as well as public figures, who tend towards authoritarianism. It should not surprise us if people with these characteristics are attracted into certain professions, notably the uniformed services and those concerned with the maintenance of the existing structure of society and the control of deviance. Indeed, a degree of authoritarianism is inseparable from the maintenance of 'law and order' as currently conceived.

PREJUDICE

Everyone is prejudiced. This book embodies the author's own class prejudices and professional prejudices, and that cannot be helped. To be prejudiced is to judge issues and people on the basis of preconceptions, and to be unwilling to be influenced by facts that do not fit in with those preconceptions (see also Chapter 26). It is always tempting to regard a person who will not accept facts as stupid; but prejudice is not the sole prerogative of people who are stupid – if by that we mean unintelligent. It has more to do with rigidity of outlook, and rigidity is itself related to the need of the individual to hold on to a world-view which is coherent and internally consistent, and the discomfort he feels when it is challenged. As a rule, rigidity increases with age.

IS BRITAIN A RACIST SOCIETY?

Certainly we have to accept that Britain is a very unequal society, in which resources and influence are in the hands of particular groups which act in their own interests and are reluctant to share power with other groups (e.g. immigrants) who are not in a position to claim it. At times this inequality becomes frank exploitation, oppression, and degradation. Xenophobia must also be admitted, and a particularly ethnocentric sense of superiority, doubtless related to Britain's geography and history. Exclusiveness and clique-distinction are certainly prevalent (whether they are getting less, and how Britain compares with other countries, are not important here). It may be that the habit of excluding people without saying why is peculiarly British and particularly difficult to overcome. When we come to authoritariansim and prejudice however, the situation is less clear. The authoritarian personality as described above would find (and does find) contemporary Britain very unsatisfactory. In the last twenty years the list of conventions that have been challenged, shibboleths abandoned, hierarchies dismantled, and moral restrictions lifted is a very long one indeed. Social inequality, acquisitive materialism, and the subordination of women have all come under fire. The public face of sexual morality has altered entirely, and the institution of marriage is under attack. Innovations in music and other arts have been bewilderingly rapid. Dress and speech are no longer the insignia of class. Hair can be worn long, short, absent altogether, or green and purple. The pace of social change is unparallelled, and appeals to tradition are greeted with derision.

Paradoxically there may be a clue here as to why racial discrimination does exist in Britain. Many, perhaps most, of the older generation of Britons are confused and disappointed by the present state of the country. They cannot understand why Britain is no longer successful and important in the world, no longer a great power. They recall a time when we 'never had it so good', society seemed orderly, secure, and destined to improve. In terms of material security this is to some extent false nostalgia; but the recollection of emotional security may be correct, in that there was more consensus about aims and moral standards, and less challenge to culturally determined value-systems. The older generation — including some who currently occupy power-bases in the social structure — are in a state of shock due to status-loss and the rapidity of social change (Toffler 1970). The changes actually have very little to do with immigration, but what could be more natural than to turn on the newcomers, who exemplify cultural difference, and use them as scapegoats? If one's own culture is breaking down, how easy to put the blame on alien intruders. The midly authoritarian person retreats into a greater authoritarianism.

Of course, this is not the whole story — exploitation has many other faces and many motives, but it is a line of approach which might, perhaps, be followed up. If, instead of shouting slogans, we can learn to recognize aspects of people's behaviour as defences against their own anxieties, we might have a more fruitful discussion. Perhaps the in-digenous Briton who stigmatizes immigrants, and the immigrant who attributes all his problems to racism, have something in common? If so, as each side retreats behind its defensive barricades, anyone who presumes to act as a mediator must expect to be shot at from both sides.

The practitioner may or may not be willing to take on the mantle of political activist, and participate in public campaigns: but at the very least we have a responsibility to ensure that our own actions and those of our professions and departments do not add to the inequalities or the exploitation. We must be prepared to speak up when necessary. Ethnic minorities do not receive equal treatment in health or social services, as examples in this book and elsewhere (e.g. Wilson 1981; Coombe 1976; Littlewood and Lipsedge 1982) clearly demonstrate. To paraphrase Friere: failure to give support to a minority does not re-present neutrality, it represents support for the majority.

THE SOCIAL PSYCHOLOGY OF MINORITY GROUPS

We must consider whether being a member of an ethnic minority is stressful, not only because of exploitation, deprivation or harassment but in the sense that the fact of group membership itself adds further psychological burdens. Elsewhere we have stated that the existence of a group to which one can belong is psychologically beneficial, whether it be an enclave group or a more diffuse one. But membership of a *despised* group has its own problems.

'People who are members of the kind of minorities with which we are concerned here share one difficult psychological problem which can be described, in its most general terms, as a conflict between a satisfactory self-realisation and the restrictions imposed upon it by the realities of membership of a minority group . . . we shall assume, both on the basis of common experience and of an endless stream of psychological studies, that it is a fairly general human characteristic to try to achieve or preserve one's self-respect and the respect of others; that it is important for most of us to have and keep as much of a positive self-image as we can manage to scrape together; and that having to live with a contemptuous view of oneself, coming from other people, constitutes a serious psychological problem.'

(Tajfel 1978 : 9)

This problem was demonstrated very neatly in a series of classic experiments using children and dolls (Clark and Clark 1939). The experiment (often repeated since, with variations) consists essentially of offering children a variety of dolls to play with, among which different ethnic groups are represented. The children are asked which they prefer, which they would like to take home, and are encouraged to make value-judgements about them (good, bad, naughty, etc.), and they are also asked to say which dolls most closely resemble themselves. The usual finding is that white children identify with white dolls and give them good attributes, while black children also tend to give good attributes to the white dolls and disparage the black ones, and have more difficulty in deciding which dolls they themselves resemble. Thus the white child is in the comfortable position where: *I am good — white doll is good — white doll is me*; but the black child's position is *I am good — black doll is bad — black doll/white doll is me?*, which is a position of *dissonance*. Post-war research in many different countries including Britain, using this and other techniques, suggests that this finding is generally true wherever there is an ethnic minority that has low status (Milner 1975). Tajfel states:

> 'This preference, shown by both groups of children, for people from one ethnic category over another represents a striking example of the acceptance by a "minority" of their status and image in the society.'
>
> (Tajfel 1978 : 12)

He comments that it is difficult to establish solid links of evidence between a child's early rejection of its own group, and any effects on subsequent attitudes and behaviour, but goes on to discuss a number of ways in which the individual might attempt to resolve such dissonances for himself, or ways in which the group itself might respond.

OPTIONS

Some sociologists list the responses to discrimination as *avoidance, aggression,* and *acceptance* (Simpson and Yinger 1953). For present purposes however we will focus on two extreme alternatives. The first is beautifully portrayed by a Caribbean poet:

Old Father

Old Father came to England in Winter '58
Cold bite him hard,
Make him bawl in his small basement room
By the Grove.
Every day he cry out:
'Man, a tekkin' de nex' boat back home'
But come spring,
Old Father still here.

Time passed.
Old Father feet begin to shift.
His roots have no meaning now.
He straighten his hair,
Press it smooth.
Coloured girls no good for he —
Day after day you see him
Bouncing down the road with a blonde,
Never brunette,
And his suit, cream or beige,
Never anything dark.

Old Father don't mix with the boys
On Saturday night no more —
No, he sit in the pub up the road —
The one at the corner
That don't like serving black people —
And he crack joke with them white people on we.
'Tut tut', he would say
'Isn't it disgusting
How they make a spectacle of themselves
At cricket matches.'

He don't say 'Hello' no more,
Don't eat dasheen or yam —
'not very digestible' —
And Heaven forbid,
He even turn his back on
Saltfish with 'chove an' dumpling.

Boy,
Old Father don't want to know we now,
In his white Rover,
With his slicked-back hair.
And them white people saying
'He's an example to his people'.

Hugh Boatswain

This does not seem to be a very 'healthy' solution, if only because the person concerned is unlikely to be fully accepted in the new group and has forfeited his place in the old. It involves so much denial as to amount almost to amputation of the past self.

At the other extreme, a psychological solution is to reject the image imposed, and set up a contradictory value-system wherein it is *we* (the minority group) who are 'good': for this to 'work' the opposition (the majority) have to be regarded as 'bad'. This is not simply a matter of disagreeing about the assessments made by the majority on the basis of its own criteria, but challenging the criteria themselves. In the case of a black-white dissonance it means rejecting the *values* that whites consider desirable: the things that blacks do, or believe, are *ipso facto* morally superior. It is not a matter of reforming the system to remove injustice. Tinkering with the system implies accepting the system — but Babylon is irredeemable. We are no longer in the business of reform, but of deliverance. Every hostile action by the 'system' reinforces the belief that Islam, or Rasta, or Zion, or whatever may be appropriate, is the one true faith and its members are the elect.

Obviously, this kind of faith can provide personal security for the individual and has done so throughout history, so long as the believer is able to ignore or reject any perceptions that cannot be fitted into the conceptual structure of the belief system. The practitioner will not wish to challenge beliefs that provide security and comfort for the individual as long as they harm no-one else: but we cannot help noticing that they lead to the formation of schisms and that in the long run seems undesirable.

The majority of members of ethnic minorities seek a compromise between these two extremes. They do not opt out of the stigmatized minority into the rest of society, nor repudiate society altogether; but remain somewhere in the middle and cope with the ambiguities. The fact that they are able to do so is, presumably, a reflection of internal security and self-evaluation strong enough to withstand external criticism and internal contradiction. The ability to live with unresolved conflicts is an attribute that we need not judge as desirable or undesirable in any moral sense, but it has something to do with what is commonly called 'stability', so on these grounds we are entitled to suggest that most members of minority groups are stable people. However, when this stability is overturned and a person becomes mentally ill, we have to remember this stress among others and take it into account.

NOTE

1   The description of the authoritarian personality has been derived largely from the critique by Brown (1965). Psychologists are usually scrupulous in keeping their descriptions value-free and avoiding the use of prejudiced terminology. In the interests of abbreviation and readability the present author has allowed those standards to slip in places and accepts responsibility for doing so.

Family Life

PRACTICAL PROBLEMS

The newcomer to Britain is obliged to make many rapid adjustments to the practical details of life. Climate is a problem for people from hot countries where it is not necessary to put on additional clothes before going out of doors, the weather is predictable from one day to the next, and a lot of domestic activity is conducted in the open air. They have to learn to have different garments for different seasons, and to be prepared to spend a good deal of money on keeping warm and dry. In warmer countries there is more social life in the streets, more gossip on doorsteps, families do not seal themselves off from each other. This applies particularly to the West Indies, but even in Pakistan where Purdah is practised, it is considerably relaxed in village society (Saifullah Khan 1976a). By contrast, having to spend one's day contained within the small confines of a terrace house in a northern city is a form of incarceration — and many women are incarcerated in that way, because they have small children to look after, or they are not permitted to go out, or they simply lack the courage to venture out into a confusing and alarming world. Similar problems affect children — a common complaint is that there is nowhere they can 'play out' unless an adult relative is prepared to take them to a nearby park.

For people from rural backgrounds, the rules of hygiene in urban settings have to be learned, including the use of dustbins and European-style lavatories. For the housewife there may be catering problems — habitual foods are either unavailable or very expensive, and she has to learn the names of acceptable English alternatives. Gas and electricity may be novelties. The list is endless. Many of the items on it are trivial, but they add up to some formidable challenges to adaptability.

ASIAN FAMILY STRUCTURE AND RESPONSIBILITIES

The extended family system traditional in villages in India and Pakistan has been described in detail by a number of authors (e.g. Saifullah Khan 1976a, 1976b, 1977, 1979; Wakil 1970; Anwar 1979). Not every Asian immigrant in Britain came from a traditional village, but the structure of the Asian family and its role-obligations is so different from the English middle-class nuclear family, and can be such a factor in the kinds of stress that are experienced and the ways they are coped with, that the practitioner dealing with any Indian or Pakistani in Britain must take it into account.

In rural India, Pakistan, or Bangla Desh, a household is likely to consist of grandparents, their married sons with their wives and children, and perhaps some unmarried or widowed sons and daughters, and other close relatives — a group of perhaps fifteen people, spanning three generations, living under one roof. The grandfather is a patriarchal figure who retains his authority however old or infirm he may be. No major decisions can be made without his approval. Property belongs to 'the family', catering is communal, housework is divided among the women under the direction and supervision of the grandmother. Meals are usually taken in two sittings, the men first and the women afterwards.

In English culture, if a young married couple are obliged to live in the home of one of their parents, this is regarded as a temporary expedient, a makeshift arrangement and a poor start for married life. An Asian family sees it quite differently. 'Two women sharing one kitchen' is not a problem, it is the norm. A newlywed couple will not have a portion of the house split off for their private use, nor be expected to spend a lot of time in each other's company, away from the rest of the household. In fact a young bride will spend more time with the other women of the house than with her husband, and her relationships with them are crucial to her happiness. She has not just married her husband, she has married *into her husband's family*, becoming a member of an existing establishment. Her position in the hierarchy will vary according to whether she has married an elder or younger son, but it is initially a fairly junior position in any case. When she has children she must still accept her mother-in-law's tutelage on their care and upbringing. If there is any dispute she cannot automatically count on her husband's support, since he is hardly more autonomous than she is as long as his father still lives (and even after his father's death he may still have to accept the jurisdiction of an elder brother).

To English eyes this hierarchical gerontocracy seems repressive and 'unfair', a negation of individual choice and self-fulfillment, but to a traditional Asian man or woman it does not appear so:

> 'He or she is not an individual agent acting on his or her own behalf . . . The individualism and independence so valued in the West appears selfish and irresponsible to a Pakistani, who expects and values the elements of dependency and loyalty . . . Family and kin take priority over individual preference.'   (Saifullah Khan 1979 : 43)

This structure, which has stood the test of time in its traditional setting, comes under strain in an urban society with geographical and social mobility. It does not work well in Karachi or Bombay. Yet most Asian immigrants to Britain have attempted to maintain or reconstruct the extended family system, and thereby hangs many a psychosocial problem.

Suppose that three brothers, each with a wife and several children, are living in Bradford or Birmingham and wish to share a house. For a start, they may have some difficulty in finding a house large enough to accomodate everyone without a degree of overcrowding that imposes strains and may offend the local authority and the neighbours. It will almost certainly be a Victorian house in a decaying area, and there may be redevelopment plans and compulsory purchase orders in the offing. Second, even if the three brothers get on well together, there is no guarantee that their wives will do so, and the grandmother who would have 'kept them in order' is not there — she is still in Pakistan. The wife of the eldest brother may try to impose her authority, but the others may not accept it. Suppose, moreover, that the younger couples under-stand English better than the elder (this is quite likely, if they all came to Britain at the same time and the younger ones spent some time in school but the eldest did not). Inevitably, the ones who speak English best and are most *au fait* with British life will take a lead in the families' dealings with the outside world — and this reversal of roles will be the more contentious if the younger ones are more 'westernized' in other ways. Even if the grandparents were present there might still be problems, because the 'oldest knows best' dictum would be contradicted: without patriarchal and matriarchal authority present, the partnership is quite likely to fall apart — causing sorrow to all concerned.

Arranged marriages

The Englishman's myths about Asian marriages are that youngsters are forced to marry whether they want to or not, the girl being not long past puberty, neither having any say in the choice of partner, having never met each other until the wedding ceremony. Arrangements are made privately between the leaders of the two families, and there is much bargaining about dowries but no-one worries about compatability of temperament or interest; family politics is all, personal happiness is unimportant.

Some of these myths may have been true of some families in India and Pakistan in the past, but they do not give an accurate picture of the usual situation in Britain today. It is true that Asians (either Hindu or Muslim) usually expect their parents to have a lot of say in their choice of partner, and very few would marry in the face of parental opposition, but it is rare nowadays that the partners have never met and know very little about each other beforehand. There is an element of political manoeuvring, in so far as every parent is looking for a 'good' match for a son or daughter — 'good' being in terms of personal prospects and/or respectable family background,[1] but few parents would knowingly sacrifice a son or daughter's happiness in pursuit of family ambition. It is also true that in rural Asia (but not in Britain) a girl would have few opportunities to meet any member of the opposite sex outside her immediate family, and therefore few opportunities to fall in love, or make comparisons. Indeed, a village girl is not expected to have strong views on any subject. From birth onwards she accepts the superior wisdom of her elders and trusts them to make right decisions for her in marriage as in everything else.

Arranged marriages have stood the test of time. Most of the Indian and Pakistani adults now in Britain had their marriages arranged for them by their parents, and most of them are happy and would not wish it otherwise. In the words of one Indian woman doctor: 'I was a young, impressionable girl, romantic and naive — if I had made my own choice I would probably have made a terrible mistake. I believed at the time that my parents were wiser than I was, and I still think that was true'. We can be quite sure, however, that her middle-class highly-educated family would have gone to a lot of trouble to find young men with whom she was likely to be compatible, would have given her some degree of choice, and certainly would not have persisted in the face of any expressed antipathy on her side or his. Among educated urban families, the system has more flexibility than the myth suggests, and this has been so for a generation or more.

The same sort of flexibility is demanded by the generation of Indian and Pakistani young men and women in Britain now approaching marriageable age. Most of them, including many of those who were born in Britain, do not wish to deny their parents any say in their marriages, but they want to be consulted. They want a compromise, and it would appear that in most families in Britain a compromise is possible, and is in fact achieved. Even with all the problems listed in this book, it seems that most Asian families in Britain are able to order their affairs to their own satisfaction, and young Asian couples are able to live happily ever after at least as often as their English counterparts.

The practitioner, however, is likely to become involved in situations where this is not the case: where a compromise is not being reached between parents and children, or a marriage is going wrong. We have to consider some of the pitfalls.

Most of the Asian parents in Britain were brought up in the kind of tradition described above, and they have the expectations and values that have been outlined. The more intelligent parents, and those who have adapted themselves to British culture, realize that traditions must change. The less intelligent, and those who stay entirely within their own community, do not. In either case their daughters are attending English schools and absorbing English values, and one of the values that the English educational system seeks to promulgate is that of thinking for oneself, having one's own ideas, developing one's own ambitions and working to fulfil them for one's own satisfaction. Teachers praise the bright child who thinks things out for herself and challenges the conventional wisdom (as long as she is reasonably polite about it). But this 'bright child' is quite different from what Pakistani parents would consider a 'good child' — obedient and deferential to her elders, demure, modest, and unadventurous. The girl can probably enact both roles quite effectively for a time, behaving quite differently at school and at home, but the crisis comes in the teens, and it is often about marriage.

To a good Muslim, British society is a moral quicksand. Islam provides a set of prescriptive and proscriptive rules for behaviour, an explicit moral code that all understand and adhere to (at least in public) and there are clear-cut sanctions against deviance. British society, on the other hand, seems irreligious and immoral. The moral code is vague and contradictory, and those who break it are not ostracized. Everyone seems to claim the right to moral self-determination, and even those whose behaviour is good seem reluctant to condemn those whose behaviour is obviously bad. The general moral decadence of Britain is demonstrated with particular blatancy in sexual matters: the permissive society is anathema.

There is, of course, a good deal of hypocrisy in Muslim moralizing about sex, as there is in Christian moralizing about sex, and it has always been the case that those who strike moral attitudes in public seldom adhere to them in private. Currently the British are becoming less hypocritical, and more open. Many would argue that this is a good thing, and that the relaxing of sexual tension and taboo has enabled a lot of other good things to happen as well, but this is not how it appears to Asian immigrants: they see rampant licentiousness all around, and they worry about its effect on their children, especially their daughters.

Many Pakistani Muslim parents have sent their daughters to Pakistan when they are approaching puberty, to preserve them from moral danger in Britain.[2] Others attempt to impose a system of chaperonage so strict that it proves counterproductive. Some have literally kept a daughter indoors throughout the entire period of time between leaving school and getting married — a degree of Purdah that is now rare in Pakistan. Others compromise, but keep a sharp eye out for any sign of misbehaviour.

In this climate of anxiety, a Pakistani girl who is seen talking to a boy at a bus stop is instantly under suspicion. The event will be reported to her parents, and will lose nothing in the telling. Then, family honour is at stake, and even the most liberal-minded parents may feel obliged to take steps to protect the family reputation, since any imputation of immorality will affect the girl's marriage prospects — and not hers alone, but her sisters' also.

The parents' fears are understandable in context, and they are not wholly unjustified. There are predatory males who hang about outside secondary schools and offer to take a girl home by car, and the naïveté of an Asian girl makes her less competent to deal with this situation than her more self-assured English classmate. There are some girls who wish to be sexually adventurous — perhaps as an act of defiance against irksome restrictions or for more universal motives. The majority, however, have no such intention. They do not seek to challenge parental authority and they do not wish to be part of the permissive society, but they find the restrictions and the prying suspiciousness of the Asian community silly and insulting and some of them rebel against it.

When confrontation occurs it often goes from bad to worse very rapidly indeed. The girl's request (whatever it was) is seen as evidence that she is already influenced by Western notions of independence. The parents are horrified. The girl is mystified and distressed — she does not wish to upset them, but what has she done wrong? They decide that they had better get her married as soon as possible. Her protestations confirm their worst fears — she must already have a boyfriend! Nothing she can say now is taken at face value. The gulf of non-communication opens wide.

This is of course an extreme and somewhat dramatized description and it does not happen in every Asian household, but it does happen sometimes and the story may end with the girl climbing out of her bedroom window and running off into the night, to turn up in due course on the doorstep of Social Services or the police station, or in a hospital casualty department after attempted suicide (Ahmed 1978; Rack 1979, 1981; Anwar and Little 1976; Ballard, C. 1979; Ballard, R. 1977).

Sexual misbehaviour by boys does not destroy family honour as much as that of girls so they are less restricted But sexual prowess is a matter of great importance and this in itself can cause problems. If an Asian youth in Britain is unable to attract a sexual partner he may develop doubts about his attractiveness. If English girls reject his advances he may attribute this to racial prejudice and become bitter. When marriage is envisaged, if he has lived many years in Britain he may reject the idea of an arranged marriage altogether, or reserve the right to reject the chosen girl once he has seen her.

Incompatibility

Muslims frequently marry cousins or other relatives; Sikhs and Hindus do not, the Hindu tradition being more concerned with caste. In both cases, however, those who arrange the marriage are concerned about compatability, and they seem to believe that this is best ensured by taking note of family background. Thus the matrimonial advertisements in Asian newspapers frequently stress 'good', or 'respectable', or 'cultured' family. Individual personality is not so much emphasized. Perhaps this does not matter if the couple are given an opportunity to appraise each other personally before the decision is made, as is normally the case nowadays, provided that both are available. Problems can arise, however, when one partner is in Britain and the other in Pakistan or India. It is not uncommon for a Pakistani father to make a trip home to seek a bride for his son among his kin, and send for the boy to come once the arrangements are made. At that stage, even if the groom does not like the look of his bride, it is difficult to cancel the arrangements. Worse, it is still possible for the girl to be brought to England for the wedding, and if it does not then take place she is in a very invidious position. She cannot remain unless she marries, and if she is sent back she arrives home in disgrace. Worse still, if her husband turns against her after the wedding has taken place, and sends her back to her family disgraced, damaged, and probably unmarriageable ever after. The same thing can happen if the bride is in Britain and the bridegroom comes to join her: but for him to return home unwed is not quite such a personal disaster.

Some of these mis-matches arise because the two partners have very different life experiences, one having lived many years in Britain while the other has never left the home village. Such differences seem to the English observer to be rather obvious: the fact that they are overlooked by the matchmakers is presumably due to the preoccupation with family rather than personal characteristics, which is itself a reflection of the Asian view of marriage as a family, rather than a personal, matter. In all these situations, it tends to be the women who suffer more than the men. If the woman has grown up in Britain and speaks English fluently, whereas her husband has just arrived and does not, it is impossible for her to behave with traditional subservience and leave all decisions to him. If she has been accustomed to going out unaccompanied and unveiled he may try to exert his authority by forbidding her to do so, and try to beat her into submission. On the other hand, a bride who comes straight from a village to join a family settled in Britain, has a double set of adjustments to make, and if her new in-laws take a dislike to her she has no-one to turn to for support. Back home, she could have sent a message to her own family, and someone would come to take up the cudgels on her behalf: in Britain she may be a Cinderella indefinitely. Not all such marriages come to an end immediately. They may go on for some time, and there may be children born before one partner finally rejects the other. Separation and divorce are always accompanied by great bitterness and recrimination, and this affects the whole family. Indeed, sometimes the marriage partners themselves disclaim responsibility, saying in effect to their relatives, 'You got me into this — you can get me out of it'.

'You are not the same person!'

For the immigrant who arrives to join other members of the family who have been in Britain for some time, or for the bride joining a husband whom she has only met in India, there may be a particular shock in store. How he (or she) has altered! He wears different clothes — carries himself differently — smokes — drinks alcohol — says things which are quite improper — neglects his religion — speaks disrespectfully of elders — is not interested in news of the family — seems to have got involved with some very dubious friends — and so on. For the newcomer, who has left behind all the familiar supports and is wholly dependent on his or her new family group, to find that they, too, have become unfamiliar — and, by implication, unreliable — is a disappointment little short of betrayal.

Nuclear interdependence

Supposing a wife is at odds with her in-laws and really unhappy, and her husband realizes this and they decide to leave his family and set up house on their own in another part of the city. Or suppose that he was in Britain on his own so the marriage is *à deux* from the outset. Does this avoid all problems? Not necessarily. Even where there is mutual affection, the nuclear family situation makes great demands. In the extended family household, personal tensions which arise are to some extent diluted by the size of the group, and the in-built role conventions. For a couple on their own, the intensity of emotional interdependence can be more difficult to cope with. Husbands do not always realize that in this situation their wives require more from them by way of companionship, affection, and shared understanding, than when they were part of a larger unit. This is particularly true if in escaping from the in-laws the couple have also escaped from the ethnic enclave, so that the wife is on her own all day with no understanding neighbours.

WEST INDIAN FAMILY STRUCTURE

The English nuclear family contains three people: mother, father and child (or children). Other people come and go (grandparents, uncles etc.) but it is the nuclear triangle that contains the strongest emotional ties and produces both stress and support. The West Indian family tends towards a different pattern. There are still three people in the nucleus but they are mother, child, and maternal grandmother. The strongest emotional ties are linear, extending through three or more generations and most influentially through the female line. A child's emotional ties to his or her father are important, but less strong than those to the mother. *Affinal* (marital) relationships are less strong than those of *lineage*: it is the 'blood line' that matters most. These differences are depicted in Figure 7(1).

Obviously, this is an oversimplified generalization, and no actual family conforms exactly to the stereotype, yet the picture of the West Indian family being kept together by the women, with husbands coming and going with casual insouciance has a certain truth in the Caribbean and in Britain. This is not to say that family ties are weak or vague. A sense of family exists in Caribbean culture as it does in Asian culture (and much more than in English culture). Obligations to brothers and sisters and others are acknowledged, and mutual support is given.

> 'Members of the household . . . offer tremendous support in times of illness . . . they seem to attach a lot of importance to each other's lives and are always willing to assist. This strong support has been especially useful in times of psychological stress and has greatly reduced the prevalence of suicides . . . suicidal fantasies are probably just as prevalent in the Caribbean as anywhere else but it appears

Figure 7(1) British and West Indian family structures

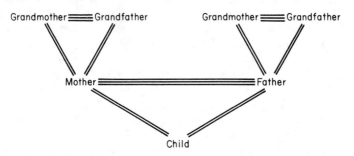

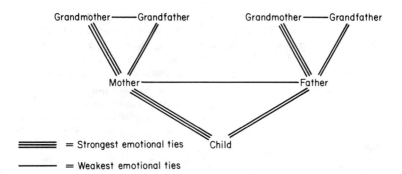

that the disgrace brought upon the family by such an act prevents
the deed.'   (Mahy 1974)

In the Caribbean Islands a child is not always looked after by its biological parents. Philpott reported that in his survey in Montserrat one
third of children were living in households in which neither parent was
present. Two-thirds were with maternal kin — commonly maternal
grandmother — and most of the others were with paternal kin (Philpott
1977). To such a child the concept of 'family' is meaningful, but the
closest bond may be with grandmother or aunt rather than mother.
This 'intra-family fostering' has a long history and one factor may be
the high rate of illegitimacy. Mahy (1974) quotes figures as high as
70–74 per cent for Granada. It is important to realize that illegitimacy
rates in the Caribbean are not the result of indiscriminate promiscuity

producing teenage pregnancies — these are indeed relatively rare. They are due to marriage being deferred until enough money and security have been acquired to set up home in a formal sense. Marriage is the seal set on a relationship, not the beginning of one. Meanwhile, if a child is born, the mother can look for support from her own mother, or aunt, or elder sister, and this family fostering or 'alternative parenting' is preferable to the problems of the single-parent family. It has been suggested that the Caribbean matrifocal family and the acceptance of pre-marital pregnancies are consequences of slavery (when marriage was forbidden):

> 'The heritage of slavery set the pattern of mating outside of marriage. The European masters were very willing to take black mistresses as is clear from the large population of mixed bloods.'

> 'The black man must break out of these irresponsible sexual patterns, and stop cluttering the islands with his illegitimate children.'

> (Mahy 1974)

Mahy writes as a black psychiatrist, but this last astringent comment seems rather unfair. These cultural patterns do not persist unchanged among the Afro-Caribbean population in Britain, but traces of them may be detected. There is less stigma attached to illegitimate pregnancy than in English society, a man does not assume that he should marry a girl whom he has made pregnant, and within marriage (or cohabitation) he does not share responsibility for home-making as most English husbands do. This attitude can seem irresponsible and feckless in the eyes of the English practitioner who does not appreciate the cultural background.

Unlike most examples of *Gastarbeiter* migration, the Afro-Caribbean immigration of the 1960s included almost as many young women as young men. Some of these women already had children, whom they left in the West Indies in the care of grandmothers or other relatives, with the intention of sending for them once the parent (or parents) were established in Britain. This led to a steady influx of children and young teenagers in subsequent years and some of these youngsters had difficulty in adapting to life in Britain because they had to adapt at the same time to a different 'parent' from those they had known so far. British Immigration Officials in the Caribbean Islands now tend to take the view that if a mother has (as they see it) 'abandoned' her child for ten years or more, she should forego the right to have the child join her in Britain. Perhaps the refusal of entry permits on those grounds is sometimes in the child's best long-term interests, but it displays an ignorance of the tradition of alternative parenting, and has caused a good deal of anger and disappointment.

A West Indian woman who has children with her in Britain suffers a particular and serious deprivation, if her own mother, to whom she would normally turn for support at times of trouble, is not available. Married or not, she may not get an equivalent amount of help from the children's father. This has been a problem for many young mothers, especially those (the majority) who have needed to remain in full-time employment. Among other things it has led to the growth of child-minding services among the Afro-Caribbean community — services which have sometimes failed to meet the standards demanded by local authorities. Another solution has been to send the child back to be brought up by its grandmother in the Caribbean. Having been born in Britain, such a child has hitherto enjoyed automatic right of return here at a later age, and the withdrawal of this right is a serious matter.

It is not, therefore, uncommon to encounter a West Indian woman (or, rather, a woman in Britain who was West Indian-born) who has never married but has several children, some of whom are in Britain and others not, and whose relationship with the children's father (or fathers) seems somewhat tenuous, while neither she nor her neighbours regard her as a loose or immoral woman. If the English practitioner can rid his or her mind of ethnocentric moral judgements they will probably discover that this woman is in no way flighty, irresponsible, or immoral, but on the contrary an extremely conscientious person coping very effectively with difficult situations.

The conventional wisdom of developmental psychology states that all children, whatever their culture, require a stable environment in their formative years, with relatively permanent adult figures of each sex with whom to identify. If this is universally true (not merely a cultural norm), it suggests that the Caribbean system of alternative parenting *as it has been practiced in the context of migration* may have been a disruptive influence in the lives of some of the young people who have grown up in one place or the other in the last twenty years, and may have contributed to the sense of alienation that some of them express.

MIXED MARRIAGES AND CHILDREN OF MIXED RACE

Given that family structure and role expectations are different between Asian, Afro-Caribbean, and WASP cultures, it is likely that people who marry 'across cultures' may have more adjustments to make than those who stay within the one culture. Their success in doing so will depend on the degree of the cultural difference and their understanding of it, the attitudes of the extended families on both sides, and situational factors, as well as their depth of affection for each other and personal characteristics. When such a couple are contemplating marriage, friends and wellwishers may wish to point out the potential difficulties, but they are not entitled to say 'It can't work', because many examples can be found in which it obviously works very well.

Batta and his colleagues have produced a series of research papers which seem to show that the children of mixed-race marriages may suffer serious disadvantages (Batta *et al.* 1965, 1980; Mawby *et al.* 1979; McCulloch *et al.* 1975). They found that while children of Asian parents had less problems than children of indigenous parents, the children of mixed parents were very much more likely to be taken into care, commit offences, and demonstrate various other symptoms of emotional disturbance and deprivation. They were, in fact, the most seriously 'at risk' of any group of children. The authors would be the first to admit, however, that these findings related to a cohort of children born at a particular place and time, and must not be extrapolated unthinkingly to mixed-parent children in general. In the initial phases of New Commonwealth migration, many of those who came were either single men, or men who had left their families behind. Not surprisingly, some of them entered into liaisons with English girls. Some of these liaisons led to marriage, others did not, and some of the marriages which took place were fairly short-lived and were superseded when the man (usually Asian) brought another woman over from the home country. At least a few of the English women who entered into such liaisons were deprived or unstable people for whom problems in marriage might have been predicted whatever their choice of partner. The offspring of such liaisons therefore in some cases started life with deprivation problems not wholly related to colour or culture. These disadvantages were later compounded by rejection from both sides, if the English mother subsequently married a white man and found her coloured children an embarrassment, but the Asian community was equally unwilling to accept them. The statistics which Batta and his colleagues discovered include many children with this kind of background. They are obviously a highly vulnerable and deprived group, whose special problems must be noted; but they belong to a particular point in the history of migration, and it would be unwise to extrapolate from this data to mixed marriages in general.

ELDERLY EXILES

Many West Indians cherish the prospect of returning 'home' on retirement, and in recent years many have done so. Pension rights are usually transferable, and the cost of living is usually less. Financial assistance with fares is also available, if required (see Chapter 23, p. 216). But many

West Indians say regretfully that they cannot go back, because there is no-one left to go back to. The rest of the family has all emigrated, if not to Britain then to America or Canada, and there are no welcoming relatives, no family property, and no-one to provide nursing care if this is eventually necessary. Asians also have the 'Myth of Return' (Dahya 1973; Anwar 1979), but the problems are similar, and most of them will remain in Britain for the rest of their lives, whether they wish to or not. Some have a specific problem regarding their supposed age. Birth certificates being unavailable in most of India and Pakistan, applicants for passports and visas have usually had to hazard a guess as to date of birth, and for various reasons some may have understated their ages; but having committed themselves, it is impossible to change. There are quite a few Asian men in Britain who look well over sixty, and from their own account feel well over sixty, and are quite unfitted to continue hard manual shift-work — but with a 'passport age' of fifty or so they are still years away from an old-age pension. In many cities there are now recognized rendezvous — perhaps a warm corner of a shopping precinct — where groups of Asian elderly men foregather to pass the time as best they can.

In theory the Asian extended family should provide a secure home and a comfortable role for the grandparent generation, and in many cases this is so. But it would be unwise to bank on the persistence of traditional values in a changed urban environment, bearing in mind all the other pressures to which the next generation is exposed. An Asian wife may not have unstinted affection for her parents-in-law (for various reasons, some mentioned above), and a sense of duty alone makes for cold charity. In the traditional rural culture, the old man retained influence right up to his death because he retained the power to apportion his property. When there is no property, but only a pension, his authority and political power within the family is diminished. So far, it seems to be true that the Asians — like the Jews before them — are able to look after their own elderly dependents. We cannot be sure that this will last.

A figure who is already present, and for whom statutory and voluntary agencies ought to be doing more than they are, is the Polish or Ukrainian widow who has been here since the war. Many of them married within their own national group, and they have children who are now grown up. Usually the husband learned to speak English in the course of his employment, but the wife did not always become completely fluent or confident. Women tend to outlive men, there are now a growing number of widows in the community, many of them living in conditions of social isolation. This isolation is bound to increase as friends die and members of the next generation become increasingly preoccupied with their own families. Adaptability decreases with advancing age. Deafness and other handicaps restrict activity. The past assumes greater importance than the future and nostalgic rumination takes the place of action. As there are less opportunities for conversation, it becomes easier to express one's thoughts (if only to oneself) in the mother tongue, so whatever level of English had been acquired starts to atrophy from lack of use, accelerated perhaps by minor strokes or the confusion of old age that affects recent memory while leaving distant memories intact. The exile is re-exiled all over again, the traumas of the refugee experience are re-lived, and emotional adjustment breaks down for the first time. Eventually she becomes unable to look after herself, and has to be looked after in a geriatric ward or old people's home. Bram (1979) has calculated that if institutional places for old people are generally required at the rate of 2.5 places per thousand population, they should be provided at a rate of seven per thousand for elderly exiles. But having been admitted to an institution her isolation is not relieved if there is no-one else there who speaks her language. Institutionalization is also, perhaps, a re-enacting of past experience: at the end of her life she becomes, once again, a refugee (Jagucki 1981; Hitch and Rack 1980).

Will this dismal picture be repeated on a larger scale in the next twenty years as the next 'generation' of immigrants arrives at old age? West Indians and Asians will not have to contend with the re-enactment of refugee traumas, but they have to live with racial prejudice and discrimination, and Asians have at least as much language difficulty as the Poles. Cold winters and expensive heating bills, which afflict all elderly people in Britain, bear particularly hard on those born in warmer climates. Now is the time for the officers of local authorities which have responsibility for provision of residential care facilities, to sit down with leaders of the ethnic minority communities and start making joint plans for the future.

ILLEGAL IMMIGRANTS

The majority of illegal immigrants are people who entered the country legally as tourists, or students, or holders of work permits for specified jobs, who overstayed their permission, and failed to take advantage of any amnesty arrangements when these were in force. Any such person is liable to be arrested, detained in custody pending investigations, and deported. He does not enjoy the legal rights of a British citizen and his case does not have to be heard in court. If he wishes to lodge an appeal before leaving the country he must make arrangements for the appeal to be lodged on his behalf by someone with authority to do so (usually a Member of Parliament). The passage of time alone does not necessarily confer the right of abode: a person may be an illegal immigrant though he has lived here openly for many years, is fully employed, and has acquired property. Some people are in this position without realizing it, and others are uncertain how they stand and unwilling to put the matter to a test.

Illegal immigrants are obviously open to exploitation. A person who comes on a work permit for a specific job becomes an illegal immigrant if he loses that job, and this gives his employer (who is the holder of the permit) the power to dictate wages and terms of service to his own advantage. If the employee changes jobs (which some do without realizing that it is illegal) he is now in a worse position, and can be bullied or blackmailed by anyone who knows the position.

It is difficult for an illegal immigrant to obtain employment through official channels, since he has no National Insurance Card or other documents (unless obtained by fraud). For the same reason he is not able to claim welfare benefits or seek assistance from statutory agencies. If such a person becomes ill, he may be afraid to seek medical treatment for fear that his presence will become known to the authorities and he will be deported. This fear is by no means fanciful. Health Service employees have already been asked to keep an eye open for persons not entitled to treatment and report those of whom they are suspicious, and some consequences of this are mentioned later.

NOTES

1   Any issue of *Dawn* or similar Indian or Pakistani newspaper will provide plenty of examples, e.g.:

'Thirty-one years Diploma Engineer all alone needs a good bride in well established family. Write Box No. . . .'

'Proposals invited from Doctors in their early thirties for a Convent-educated fair-complexioned Lady Doctor in her mid twenties. Contact with full details Box No. . . .'

'From only well placed cultured families with background compatible match for Sunni dynamic bank officer 26, U.P. family, fair complexion essential. Details to Box No. . . .'

'Suitable match for late thirty gentleman well placed in England well educated on short visit here seeks suitable match fair complexioned lady 20–30. Write in confidence to Box No. . . .'

Note as well as the stress on family respectability, the importance of fair complexion.

2   In the schools of Bradford and parts of Birmingham where a significant
    number of the pupils are Asian, it is quite noticeable that although in the
    younger classes there are approximately equal numbers of boys and girls,
    higher up the school the boys remain but there are few girls.

Identity

PROBLEMS ARE NOT NECESSARILY CULTURAL

On first meeting a patient or client whose cultural or racial background might be significant, the practitioner will wish to ask whether his client was born in Britain, and if not, at what age did he or she first arrive. As a matter of courtesy this question ought not to be asked at the very outset, but it is an important question that has to be introduced into the conversation, because at the present time there are adolescents and young adults who were born in Britain of immigrant parents, and there are others of similar age who have only recently arrived. The cultural factors mentioned already, and in Part III, apply mainly to the recent arrivals, and a person who has been brought up entirely in Britain will be justifiably offended if he or she is automatically assumed to be a newcomer.

As a simple rule of thumb, the important watershed is the school leaving age, sixteen. The longer a person was in Britain before reaching that age, the more they were exposed to the cultural, as well as the educational, influences of the school environment.

The point is illustrated by three sisters in the same family, now aged twenty-five, twenty-one, and seventeen, who arrived from Pakistan eight years ago with their mother to join their father and brothers already here (a not uncommon story). The eldest never attended school in Britain, speaks little English, and has no wish to challenge the cultural assumptions of her parents. The youngest started school here at the age of nine, speaks fluent English, has a clear understanding of British culture, and may have quite different ambitions. The middle one is an intermediate — and perhaps more difficult — position. None of them are in the situation of the person of similar age who was born in Britain of parents who long ago made the decision to become settlers here and have already come to terms with most of the cultural ambiguities in their own lives.

Disputes between parents and adolescent children are a normal feature of family life and are not necessarily connected with culture. Ahmed (1981) has an important warning against using the concept of 'culture conflict' to explain all problems. But even if the dispute is not related to culture, background 'material' can be used as ammunition, e.g.:

'Don't keep telling me about Poland, I'm not interested.'

'You let them walk all over you — that's why they despise us.'

'I don't understand you when you talk Punjabi — that's Paki talk — speak in English — why are you so ignorant?'

'Why you always try copy them, they laughing at you — you never tell us about black history, never give us a thing to be proud of.'

'They always talk Vietnam, Vietnam, Vietnam, and crying. Vietnam was *bad* place.'

'I am not West Indian. You are — but I am a Black Britisher!'

(All statements heard by, or reliably quoted to, the author)

The point need not be laboured here, as examples of conflict and distress in the relations between ethnic minority youth and parents, and between youth and the rest of society, are mentioned in many other chapters. The educational resources which ought to be made available for this section of the population are well documented elsewhere, and are outside the scope of this book. So is the vexed question of the relationship between the police and the Afro-Caribbean community. These are both extremely important matters and practitioners who take seriously their commitment to ethnic minorities ought to keep abreast of events affecting 'race relations' generally.[1]

In recent years young adults born in Britain of Asian parents have started to protest against condi˙ ɔns here by taking political action — either forming ethnic political parties, or joining existing political groups (usually among the radical left). They are more active in British politics than their parents, and relatively uninterested in the politics of India or Pakistan. Young adults with West Indian parents, on the other hand, although just as dissatisfied with Britain, are less politically organized here but more interested in the politics of the Caribbean than their parents are. These are, of course, crude generalizations to which there are many exceptions, but they indicate that there are several possible reactions to the same predicament. The situation is changing so rapidly that a description of any particular group or tendency is immediately out of date; but as a case in point the Rastafarian movement is significant and ought to be more widely understood.

RASTAFARI

The history of Rastafari begins in the early years of this century with a Jamaican activist, Marcus Garvey. Garvey set out to unify black Jamaicans with an appeal that was both political and religious. His doctrine was millenarian — i.e. looking to a time of deliverance in the future when his oppressed people would come into their inheritance. He saw this in terms of a return to Africa, and organized various unsuccessful 'repatriation' schemes. His most famous directive to his followers was to 'look to Africa when a black King shall be crowned, for the Day of Deliverance is near'. Such an event occurred in Ethiopia in 1930 when Prince Ras Tafari ascended the throne as the Emperor Haile Selassie, and although by then Garvey was something of a spent force, his followers saw this as the sign they had awaited.

For people brought up on the scriptures the comparison between their situation and the old testament history of the captivity of the Jews was appealing, and the Rastafari came to see themselves in that light, and adapted scriptural descriptions and prophecies to their own situation. Thus their God became *Jah*, or *Jah-Jah*. Ethiopia became *Zion* and their place of captivity *Babylon*. By a series of associations supported by selective use of scriptural texts, *Ethiopia* has come to be the name for the whole of Africa; *Babylon* is everywhere else, and is not only a place but a name for the condition of black servitude in white society.

One characteristic of the Rastafari is to allow their hair to grow long and plait it in 'locks'; another is the use of marihuana (cannabis) variously known as *ganja*, hash, or 'the herb'. Until the last twenty-five years the 'Rastas' in Jamaica were regarded as harmless eccentrics. Various researchers emphasized the pacifism of the movement and the reasonable desire of its members to improve their squalid living conditions, and some supported their request to be 'repatriated' to Africa (echoing Garvey's earlier plea, with as little success). In the 1950s however, gross social inequalities and increasing deprivation in Trenchtown and other slums of Kingston produced physical as well as verbal violence, and this in turn provoked a repressive Government reaction. By this time the movement had attracted some support from Jamaican students who injected a sharper ideology of social revolution. A movement which was previously comparable with the 'Hippie' or 'Flower People' cults started to acquire a harder edge of social and racial protest.

Jamaica remains the centre of the movement, but there are groups of

'Rastas' in most other Caribbean islands. In Dominica a law was passed against long hair. In St Lucia the Rastas are credited with having caused a change of government in 1979. In Barbados they are said to steal from gardens (on the grounds that all plants belong to *Jah* and therefore to everyone) and pilfer from tourists. In fact 'Rasta' has become a term applied by the 'establishment' in the Islands to any group of young people who have long hair and are thought to be antisocial, whether they subscribe to the millenarial doctrines of Marcus Garvey or not. Much the same thing has happened in Britain. Because some of the young, politically minded activists in the black community have adopted the Rasta identity, and their appearance (especially the long hair) is a challenge to the official image of what a respectable, law-abiding young person should look like, the police do tend to regard them as potential trouble-makers. The association with cannabis is also held against them.

There is a sense in which the establishment is quite right to regard Rasta as a threat. Any movement — religious or secular — that preaches radical reform and rejects the current values of society must be a threat to the status quo, especially if it provides a sense of identity and group cohesion for a sizeable, active, and alienated section of the population. But it is a mistake to regard all Rastas as antisocial, anti-White, drug-taking delinquents. No doubt some are, and have merely jumped on the bandwagon with no idea of the underlying philosophy of the movement. For others it is a religion, and provides the support, consolation, and sense of purpose that religions traditionally provide for their followers: its tenets are brotherhood, openness, love to all, and rejection of materialism. If *deliverance from oppression* is a religious concept and *resistance to oppression* is a political one, Rasta would seem to be more religious than political. Reggae music, and the songs of Bob Marley in particular, illustrate both the anger and the idealism of Rasta, and are an important source of inspiration. For many British Rastas the history of Marcus Garvey is now irrelevant; the movement is still about black brotherhood, and Africa may still be used to symbolize that, but the problems are here, within society. Rasta is concerned with consciousness-raising, about changes between people that depend on changes *within* people. The following prose-poem, written by a member of a Sheffield youth club in 1981, expresses this:

Babylon System

> BABYLON is not just the police, but everything
> that dwell within the system, that is how I see
> it. The system is Babylon, all they want is an
> easy way to obtain money and riches, and so become
> well-known. They system is there to oppress

the people in becoming the way they are, forcing
them away from the truth.
BUT I and I dwell not in Babylon, for their ways
are not I man ways. They seek darkness, I seek
light.
BABYLON is everywhere, in the city, in the country,
in men and women. The only way of escaping
Babylon is to seek the most High God and your
soul shall be free from the open mouths of the
wicked.
BABYLON comes in many forms, your mother, father,
sister, friend, anyone, but trying to explain
Babylon would take I man for ever. But there is
one word that says it all — EVIL. All a one can
do is fight it with the power of Jah, for Jah
will protect his children from all the evil
men.

(from Finding Me, Hub Publicatons 1981)

(The biblical flavour of the language, and the distinctive usages I-and-I, and I-man, are characteristic of Rasta speech.)

Rasta provokes hostility not just among whites but as much, if not more, from the older generation of West Indians in Britain. In Britain, though not in the West Indies, it is an exclusively young person's movement. It is, perhaps, a characteristic of teenagers and young adults that they are able to discuss their views and feelings with each other with a frankness and trust that, all too often, older people seem to lack. This is as true of West Indian youth as it is of Anglo-Saxon youth, and perhaps more so. Naturally the practitioner (if an outsider) cannot expect to be admitted to these discussions, but he should not underestimate their importance. Some of the discussions that take place in Rasta groups (the term used is 'reasonings') take on the character of group psychotherapy, and provide something in the lives of participants which may go far beyond the superficial comfort of 'club membership'.

NOTE

1 The Runnymede Trust publishes a regular *Bulletin* of background, factual and statistical information and the Journal *'New Community'* contains relevant articles. At local level the Community Relations Councils may welcome support from practitioners (see Appendix 5).

Breakdown

Culture and Concepts of
Mental Illness

Because of all the stress already mentioned we might suppose that minority groups would all have high rates of mental disorder. This is not the case, but statistics can be misleading unless they are interpreted carefully. A person who is distressed or cannot cope only becomes a psychiatric patient (and therefore a statistic) if he or she produces symptoms that are not only abnormal but fall into the particular category that society and the medical profession choose to call 'illness'. One person responds to stress by drinking too much, another by smoking too much. The first may figure in the statistical returns of either psychiatrist or probation officer, the second in neither. This is within one culture — when we look across cultures we find much greater differences, firstly in the *manifestations* of distress, and secondly in the *interpretations* of those manifestations.

When a member of an ethnic minority develops a mental illness, the manifestations *may* be very much the same as in the familiar British-born patient.[1] If so, once communication problems have been overcome, treatment can be given along familiar lines. But they *may* be different, and then there is a danger of misdiagnosis and wrong treatment. The similarities outweigh the differences, but it is the differences that concern us.

For example: a middle-aged Pakistani woman in Bradford began to behave coquettishly towards her husband, and then towards other men in the household. When rebuked, she expressed with some vehemence her right to have opinions of her own, and said that if her husband disliked her behaviour he could leave her. This forthright speech convinced all her relatives that she had gone mad, and they brought her to a psychiatrist. The doctors and nurses, who were English, found no evidence of mental illness. She appeared to them to be a rather jolly, extravert, uninhibited person, but nothing more. It required a psychiatrist who understood the norms of Pakistani culture to point out that her lack of decorum was highly unconventional in that cultural context, and probably due to hypomania.

Conversely, a person may behave in ways which seem odd or bizarre to the practitioner, and lead him to suppose that mental illness is present, when in fact the behaviour is culturally normal or explicable.

Another possibility is that all the parties agree that something unusual is occurring, but they do not necessarily regard it an *illness*. Suppose, for example, that in some part of Africa a hitherto normal man begins to behave in odd unpredictable ways. His relatives may suspect that he is *possessed by a spirit*. Suppose they take him to the local healer, who examines him carefully and agrees that he is indeed *possessed*. As soon as that has been said, the victim is relieved for the time being of normal social obligations. He receives sympathy. He is not obliged to work. If his behaviour is anti-social he escapes retribution, since the blame is not with him but with the *evil spirit*. If it is necessary to restrain him forcibly this is done without rancour. After observing the victim and listening to the account given by his companions, the medicine man *identifies the evil spirit* and instructs how it should be placated or driven out. The process involves performing various rituals and swallowing certain compounds, and also some changes of habits — removal to a different house, perhaps, or carrying out some neglected obligations either *by* the victim or by someone else *to* him. If the medicine man is good at his job and correctly identifies the evil spirit, the victim is relieved and becomes normal.[2]

In Britain on the other hand, if a man starts to behave in odd unpredictable ways, his relatives say — he must be *ill*. They take him to the psychiatrist at the local hospital, who examines him and says that he is indeed *ill*. When that has been said, the patient is relieved for the time being of normal social obligations. He receives sympathy. He is not obliged to work. If his behaviour is anti-social he escapes retribution, since the blame is not with him but with his *illness*. If it is necessary to restrain him forcibly this is done without rancour. After observing the patient and taking a detailed history, the psychiatrist *makes a diagnosis* and prescribes treatment. This may include a variety of therapies and psychotropic drugs and also some changes of habits — a different job, perhaps, or reappraisal of some personal relationships and conflicts. If the psychiatrist is good at his job and has correctly diagnosed the illness, the patient is relieved and becomes normal.

The conceptual model is different, but in this case it does not seem to make much difference to treatment. We may want to ask, however, did the African healer really believe that the patient was possessed by a spirit, his mind and body invaded by an alien entity? Or did he recognize that the man was having problems with his mother-in-law, and needed a way of getting her out of the house? Was 'possessed-by-an-evil-spirit' merely a figure of speech?

The same question can be addressed to the psychiatrist. If he derives his metaphor — 'illness' — from a medical rather than a religious source, is it any less a metaphor? This is a sensible question. Before answering it, most British psychiatrists would probably wish to make a distinction between *psychoses* and *neuroses*. Psychoses do have some of the characteristics of 'diseases' — including biological as well as psychological concomitants: the medical model fits them reasonably well. Neuroses do not fall so easily into that model, and perhaps ought not to be forced into it: for them, perhaps the word 'illness' is a kind of metaphor (Torrey 1974 : 139). The distinction between the two can be overstated, and does not always stand up to close scrutiny, but in practice clinicians tend to adopt a more 'biological' stance towards psychoses (for example, manic/depressive psychosis or schizophrenia), and a more 'psychological' stance towards neuroses (for example, hysteria and anxiety states). We shall start from this orthodox position and envisage a continuum of mental disorders, with the more 'biological' at one end and the more 'psychological' at the other. We shall find, however, that cultural differences oblige us to modify this concept as we go along. (For the benefit of non-psychiatrist readers, Appendix 1 contains a brief guide to psychiatric terminology and classification.)

Cultural differences in the manifestations of distress and the way such manifestations are interpreted, represent *diagnostic pitfalls* for the practitioner, and are considered as such in the next five chapters. We have to consider whether a familiar illness (such as endogenous depression) has a different presentation in different cultures; or, to put the same question the other way round, whether a familiar symptom has a different meaning in different cultures.

Suppose, for example, that a patient complains of headache. Then suppose that he goes on to say that his headache is caused by an enemy who is employing Black Magic against him. If this were a well-educated indigenous patient the doctor might well find the explanation bizarre, and start to suspect a paranoid psychosis. But in pre-scientific societies such beliefs are commonplace (see Chapters 4 and 20), and the only safe conclusion is that the patient has a headache and is worried. The complaint cannot be ignored: the patient has, after all, a problem (the headache) that requires investigation. There are various possibilities:

(1) His headache may have a simple physical cause, and the fact that he says unexpected things about it is irrelevant.

(2) His headache (with a simple physical cause) may be worrying him so much that he has developed an *anxiety state* about it, and he is expressing his anxiety in a culturally normal way.

(3) He may have an anxiety state for some quite different reason, and the anxiety may be causing his headache. It is possible that his anxiety may be connected with (for example) a family quarrel: and in that case if he says that a relative is causing his headache he is quite right.

(4) His fears about magic, and his headache, may both be due to a paranoid or depressive psychosis.

The choice of treatment will depend on which of these alternatives the practitioner selects. He has to find his way through a diagnostic maze. If there is no physical cause for the headache it must be, by definition, 'mental'. So the term 'mental illness', it seems, must cover everything from *worry* to *madness* — from legitimate anxiety to florid psychosis.

This is more than a little confusing to laymen, and indeed to professionals,[3] and never more so than when we are working across cultures. We have to assess abnormal behaviour against a background which is itself unfamiliar, taking note of two kinds of difference at once. We must take particular care not to diagnose someone as mentally ill simply because he is out of step with society: 'If a man does not keep pace with his companions perhaps it is because he hears a different drummer. Let him step to the music he hears, however distant' (Thoreau 1817–62, *Walden*).

NOTES

1 A semantic problem has to be acknowledged here. Asians and West Indians in Britain are of course British, and their cultures however distinctive are British cultures. No contrary implication is intended: but we do need to be able to make comparisons by referring to *the indigenous patient whose culture and habitual behaviour is already familiar to the practitioner*, and to use so lengthy a phrase each time would be tedious.

2 Accounts similiar to this may be found in, for example, Torrey (1972); Obeyesekere (1969); Lewis (1971).

3 Several authorities who have tackled the problem of defining the boundaries of mental illness have ended up by concluding that illness is 'what doctors treat'. See for example, Kraupl Taylor, Linder, and others cited in Kendall (1975). Kendall discusses the validity of psychiatric classification in considerable detail. See also Kessell (1965); Torrey (1974); Wallace (1961, Chapter 6); Laing (1960, 1967); Laing and Esterson (1964); Szasz (1961, 1971); Cox (1976); Leff (1981); Murphy (1982).

Cultural Pitfalls in the Recognition of Depression and Anxiety

SOMATIZATION

A familiar psychiatric patient is the middle-aged woman who complains of depression. She looks miserable, weeps readily, has lost interest and concentration, sleeps badly and wakes early, feels hopeless about the future, and blames herself for her own condition. These features are suggestive of *endogenous depression* (see Appendix 1) and as well as the mental and emotional complaints, she probably has backache, diffuse muscular aches and pains, and a sense of general weariness and lassitude.

An Indian or Pakistani woman with the same condition will usually complain of pain and weakness. The pain may be in the back, limbs, or head, or diffused throughout the body (best described as 'body ache'). Discomfort in the chest or abdomen is particularly common, and she may say that there is gas in her body which comes up into her head. The weakness is generalized, described in terms 'I have lost all my strength'. If the patient were a man, he might also mention sexual dysfunction. Often the patient has his or her own ideas on causation, and complains that there is something wrong with the heart, liver, or bowels.

If we ask the right questions we may be able to elicit feelings of unhappiness and the other features of the depressive syndrome: but the *presentation* is different. The British-born woman described her mood first, and her somatic symptoms as an afterthought or only on questioning: the Indian or Pakistani patient did it the other way round. Indeed, she might not admit to the depressed mood at all — which puts the practitioner in the position of diagnosing 'depressive illness' *without any apparent depression.*[1]

Somatization of emotional distress applies to depression (whether endogenous or reactive) and to anxiety. It is by no means unknown among the indigenous British, especially the less articulate and the elderly. It is very well recognized by clinicians in India (Carstairs 1958a, 1975; Rao 1966; Neki 1973), Pakistan (Mubbashar 1977; Bavington 1981), Bangla Desh (Chowdhury 1966; Rahman 1970), Hong Kong (Kleinman 1977), the West Indies[2] and various parts of Africa.

> 'Among African patients somatic symptoms play a major, predominant role, and they tend to push psychological symptoms into the background.'   (Adomakoh 1975)

> 'Hamilton's triad of depressed mood, guilt and suicide should be modified (in African cultures) to read: depressed mood, projected guilt, suicide *and multiple bodily complaints.'*   (Binitie 1975)

(See also Leighton *et al.* (1963))

The West Indian idiom however, can be confusing: a patient may say he has 'low feelings' but this is a reference to physical lassitude and debility, not state of mind.

The uninitiated clinician is easily led astray by somatization. If he is too much impressed by physical symptoms, and orders unnecessary investigations, X-rays, and specialist referrals, this merely confirms the patient's own belief that there is some physical disorder, and makes eventual psychiatric diagnosis more difficult. Alternatively, having failed to discover any cause the practitioner shrugs it off as 'hypochondriasis'. Hypochrondriasis is not a diagnosis: it is a symptom — maybe of depression, anxiety, hysteria, or something else — which requires to be followed up.

Why would the Pakistani patient complain of the somatic aspects of the condition, and omit (perhaps even deny) the emotional ones? We may explain it in various ways. At the simplest level it may relate to beliefs about *what a doctor is for.* British patients have learnt about depression, anxiety, and so on and they realize that these may have medical causes and can be discussed directly with doctors. Most Asians do not go to doctors unless they have something physical to mention, since in their view that is the province of doctors. If an Asian person experiences 'pure' emotional distress, with no somatic accompaniments, he or she usually tries to sort it out within the family, or seek help from some other, *non-medical* source. Indian clinicians report that although 'depression' is well enough recognized when the right questions are asked in community surveys it is rare as a cause of medical consultation. Similar reports have been made in Africa and elsewhere.

A second alternative explanation is that the somatic complaint is a metaphor. A British patient might say that he had a 'lump in the throat, or 'butterflies in the tummy', or a depressed patient might say that he was 'heartbroken' (Leff 1973, 1977, 1981). Similarly in Urdu a common description of distress is *'mera dil dukta'* (*dil* = heart); but a patient who says this does not expect to be referred to a cardiologist and is usually the first to recognize that a mistake has been made if this happens — which it does from time to time. In his research on Hakims (Asian traditional healers) Aslam (1979) noted that a lot of patients gave vivid descriptions of their 'heart distress':

> 'The symptoms were described . . . as "My heart is sinking" or "fluttering" (*Dil thadakdah hey*); "My heart feels lonely, squeezed, bored" (*Dil paereshan hey*). The patients illustrated these by first pounding on the chest, or hand squeezing to illustrate a "pressed heart" . . . *Frequent expressions included* "My heart gives me news" (*Mera dil kabitah hey*) — said of a premonition; "My heart burns" (*Mera dil saddtha hey*) said when describing a tragic event.'
>
> (Aslam 1979 : 129)

In the diagnostic techniques of Hakims great importance is attached to the pulse, and this may be the reason why palpitations are defined as an illness. At the same time, Aslam states that in Muslim culture the heart provides 'an idiom for expressing emotion', and it was apparently so regarded by the Hakim:

> 'The Hakim in these circumstances also described the ailment more as physical sensations associated with a particular feeling of anxiety. Particular emphasis was placed on the reasons for the anxiety which caused the heart discomfort. This symptom was mainly exhibited in females more than in males. The Hakim stressed that this was an illness of women who had migrated to England from their extended families in Asia. The main reasons given by the women were sorrow, worry, anxiety . . . typically arising from a death in the family, leaving behind relatives in Asia, disagreement with sister-in-law or mother-in-law or spouse.'   (Aslam 1979 : 130)

An English-speaking patient might experience the somatic manifestations of anxiety and describe them in roughly similar manner, but would also be able to refer directly to the emotional experience without relying on metaphor because more specific words are available to them. In many Asian and African languages, even if specific words are available, the somatic metaphor is the customary means of expression.

A third possibility is that the physical symptoms are the only ones which are acceptable to the patient. A clear example of this is provided by Kleinman:

> 'Mr. H . . . would tell me that he was depressed, but then describe that in somatic terms. If I asked him about his personal feelings he

would not tell me anything other than that he was getting better. He would tell me repeatedly that his financial problems caused his sickness (which he believed to be a physical disorder) but if I asked him how this made him feel, tears would come to his eyes, which his facial muscles would strain to hold back, and he would look away for minutes at a time. He would tell me that these were things that were better not talked about, that he never talked about them with anyone, *even with himself*, that after all they were getting better; and then he would politely but firmly introduce another topic. Even after four months, when his depression had largely subsided, Mr H . . . refused to talk about what his feelings had been like. In fact, on one occasion he told me that he himself did not know what they were like since when they came to mind he felt his somatic symptoms greatly worsen and became preoccupied with the latter.'
(Kleinman 1977 : 7)

This example is from Hong Kong. Kleinman explains that mental illness carries a great stigma among the Chinese. Therefore only indisputably psychotic behaviour is labelled as 'mental illness' by them. Minor psychiatric problems are commonly labelled as medical illnesses, or rather, the somatic aspects are labelled as medical, while the psychological issues are 'systematically left unlabelled'. Not all Chinese clinicians agree with this (Yap 1965) but it fits very well with our own experience with Indian and Pakistani villagers in Britain, for whom 'mental illness' has a similar stigma. Somatization in this case is a psychological defence mechanism. By emphasizing the somatic aspects the subject places himself *in his own estimation* in the category 'ill' rather than in the category 'mad'. Kleinman's example demonstrates that this may not be deliberate: his patient *could not bring himself* to contemplate his own emotional distress and found that whenever he tried to do so his somatic symptoms became worse and dominated his consciousness. We can regard this as an hysterical manouevre, no different from any other hysterical patient who 'converts' some unacceptable internal conflict into physical symptoms (though Kleinman himself does not make this point). Even if this only applies in a few cases it is a useful insight: to turn the example round, it suggests that when we have diagnosed a patient as hysterical, and are seeking underlying causes, we should include a depressive illness — or rather, the stress of having a culturally unacceptable depressive illness — among the possibilities. British psychiatrists and psychiatric nurses are apt to see hysteria and depression as opposed — the more hysterically a person acts, and the more somatic ailments he produces, the less they are convinced of the 'genuineness' of his depression — so this is a real diagnostic pitfall when it occurs.

Separately or in combination, these three factors may be sufficient to explain why many non-Europeans tend to somatize their emotional distress, and why reports on the incidence of depression in various cultures are unreliable. For the practitioner, the important point to remember is that depression or anxiety may well be the correct diagnosis even if emotional symptoms are specifically denied. But this is not necessarily the whole story: it is instructive to use the issue of somatization to explore some other possible connections between illness, emotion, race, and culture.

THE PERCEPTION AND INTERPRETATION OF SUBJECTIVE EXPERIENCE

So far, we have assumed that the subjective experience of distress is the same in all cultures: it has both mental and physical aspects, and people differ only in those that they choose to emphasize. We must consider the alternative possibility that people do not all experience the same emotions.

The early European investigators who made forays into the exotic worlds of Africa and elsewhere reported that 'primitive' people were incapable of experiencing the depths and subtleties of emotion known to the white races. The mind of the 'primitive' functioned — it was believed — at a cruder level. The feelings of the 'native' were like those of a child, or else — in one memorable comparison — like a white man leucotomized. 'Primitive' behaviour was the result of 'primitive' mental processes in 'primitive' brains. Starting from those premises, psychiatrists were not surprised to find that depression seemed to be rare in 'primitive' cultures: melancholy and despair were the prerogative of civilized urban man, not the 'noble savage', the simple 'child of nature', or the 'lesser breed'.[3]

This view has been found offensive by most later investigators. The 'primitive brains' idea has not been upheld by scientific investigation, and it now seems academically disreputable to make comparisons between races on the grounds of their supposed biological limitations. The current view is that even if the brain is not absolutely identical the world over, it is so nearly identical that differences pale into insignificance beside the effect of culture and environment.[4] In this climate of opinion there has been a tendency to look for similarities rather than differences. Post-war studies have usually shown that depressive illness exists wherever it is looked for, if the questions are rightly framed.

In this discussion there are actually two arguments going on at the same time. One is about the incidence of depressive illness (using that term to imply a biological substrate); the other is about the capacity of individuals to experience emotions. These are different arguments, since of all the people who experience a depressed mood only a few are suffering from a depressive illness — and conversely it is possible to have a depressive illness without much in the way of mood disorder. Since endogenous depression does have some genetic aspects, it is quite possible that its prevalence varies in genetically different groups, exactly as do diabetes and several other disorders: if we can get rid of the offensive condescension of the 'primitive brains' notion we can keep an open mind about differences in prevalence. But even if we found somewhere a group (or race) that was totally immune from depressive illness, that would not say anything about the capacity of those people to experience emotions. The two questions are linked only in so far as the experience of depression is an important component of depressive illness, and if it does not seem to be present the diagnosis is more difficult. To do justice to the complexities of this it would be necessary to make a metaphysical digression into the nature of experience. Two points, however, are worth making. Kleinman (among others) has pointed out that an experience of any kind includes not only what is happening *to* you (or *in* you) but what you make of it. What is experienced is not just 'depression' but the subject's own interpretation of it. The premenstrual tension syndrome provides a useful illustration. A woman who becomes emotionally unstable during the premenstrual week usually feels quite differently about it as soon as she recognizes the association. She may still be upset, but if she can blame it on her hormones she no longer has the added burden of being upset *about being upset*. She has an explanation about her feelings and can cope with them better. In West Africa, women who are depressed commonly say that they have become witches. The idea of witches is culturally valid, and in fact rather commonplace, (Kiev 1972). To object that hormones exist but witches do not is to miss the point: if the explanation is culturally valid and not in itself shameful, it can be used to rob the experience of some of its mystery. The interpretation of the experience alters the quality of the experience itself.

LINGUISTIC FACTORS

The second point involves a digression into the field of linguistics. The English language is extremely rich in words to describe mood states. In addition to 'depressed' one can be despondent, despairing, disconsolate, dispirited, disillusioned, gloomy, melancholy, miserable, morbid, morose, unhappy, sad, and so on. Not all these words are in daily colloquial use, but most reasonably articulate English speakers will use some of them and recognize others. They are not exactly synonyms, but seem to have fine shades of meaning. Statements like 'He is *sad* about the death of his dog, but he is not letting it make him *miserable*'; or 'Are you *depressed*?' 'No, but I am *unhappy*', seem to be meaningful, even if we would be hard-pressed to define the exact meanings. In many non-European languages, however, no such vocabulary exists. In Yoruba, for example, one word suffices for both 'angry' and 'sad' — two emotions that most Europeans would consider to be quite distinct. In Ghana three words cover all shades of unpleasant emotion: one of them refers primarily to the somatic accompaniments and another implies 'hurt' — i.e. inflicted. Similar restrictions apply in many other African languages, and perhaps the best English translation is the equally ambiguous 'upset'.

Rather than feel superior about our 'rich' vocabulary we should reflect on some of our own limitations. In family relationships, for example, the phrase '*brother-in-law*' is ambiguous: it may refer to *wife's brother*, or *sister's husband*, or even perhaps to *wife's sister's husband*. These are quite different relationships, which in most family-centred cultures would have quite different role obligations and merit different words. Similarly, a *cousin* is notoriously vague in English — it does not even differentiate gender. The old distinction between *Gran* and *Nan* (paternal and maternal grandmother) persists in dialect only.

We may take this as a hint — if nothing more — that in contemporary British culture the accurate distinction of different relationships does not merit high priority: whereas our plethora of introspective words suggests that we are fascinated, preoccupied, obsessed even by our own internal experiences. Rather than say that some languages are 'primitive', we should conclude that each culture develops a rich vocabulary around the issues which seem particularly important to those people at that time. Laplanders allegedly have over twenty different words for snow — presumably because snow which is soft or crisp, old or fresh, static or drifting, is different, and the differences are important and must be made specific.

If this formulation is correct, there will obviously be difficulties in translation, and in our experience it is often quite pointless to ask an Urdu speaker whether his feelings are mainly those of *anxiety* or of *sadness*. Yet a great deal of psychiatric diagnosis depends heavily on just such a question.[5]

This digression into linguistics leads us back to our intitial question: is the *experience* the same even if the vocabulary is different? If the only available word is 'upset' is the experience equally non-specific? Does the Pakistani not know whether he is anxious or miserable? Are Nigerians always angry when they are sad and vice versa? Obviously not. But we must recognize that vocabulary not only serves to record and communicate experience, but also focuses, verifies, and to some extent alters it (Boaz 1940). Berger, writing about inarticulate sections of the English middle and working class, says: 'They are deprived of the means of translating what they know into thoughts which they can think . . . a great deal of their experience — especially emotional and introspective experience, has to remain un-named for them' (Berger and Mohr 1967 : 98–9). Another way of expressing this is the Sapir-Whof formulation, which is a well-known (though not undisputed) principle of linguistics: 'language functions not merely as a means of reporting experience but also, and more significantly, as a way of defining experinece' (Hoijer 1974 : 121). This brings us back to the issue of somatization. In order to make a distinction between distress in the mind and distress in the body, and describe each one separately, it is necessary to recognize a clear dichotomy between the concepts 'mind' and 'body'. Such a dichotomy, though tacitly accepted in European thought, has no inherent validity nor can it claim universal acceptance. An earlier statement about this was: 'the primitive not only does not separate the diseases of the body and mind in his medical concepts, but does not recognize such separate units' (Ackernacht 1948). This statement appears to be the same: but it is in fact slightly different because it occurs in the context of the 'primitive brains' school of thought, with the implicit assumption: 'these people are *inherently incapable of . . .*'. Our explanation is in terms of cultural priorities. As Leff points out, any Englishman would be capable of appreciating the different types of snow that the Laplander describes, but 'until his eyes are opened to the differentiation and its practical implications, the Englishman will go on seeing all the different varieties of snow as one indivisible continuum' (Leff 1973).

In many non-European cultures (including those of rural Asia) people derive their sense of identity, their self-concepts, to a large extent from their roles and positions in society, and their interactions with others. They are less accustomed to visualize themselves in terms of what is happening inside their own heads.

If language serves to chart an experience introspectively, then it is at least possible that the internal experiences concerned in 'depression' are modified by the words available. Our two depressed patients (English and Pakistani) may be having similar emotional experiences, but we cannot be sure that they are identical.

GUILT

Guilt is an important diagnostic feature of depressive illness in Western society. We expect the depressed patient to say that he or she is a burden on others, has done wrong, and perhaps does not deserve to live. Some are tormented by a sense of their own unworthiness or wickedness, and give accounts of misdeeds which may be exaggerations of trivialities in the past, or even frankly delusional. Psychiatrists generally attach a lot of importance to this symptom in assessing the 'genuineness' and severity of the depression, and estimating the risk of suicide.

Yet guilt is to some extent a culture-bound concept. It has been said that there are 'guilt-based societies' and 'shame-based societies'. The distinction will not stand very close scrutiny but is useful up to a point. A guilt statement is 'I have done something wrong, and even if it is never discovered, and nobody else but me knows about it, I am distressed and disgusted with myself, and cannot overlook it'. A 'shame' statement would be: 'I have done something wrong in the eyes of other people. People who matter to me are disgusted with my behaviour, and therefore I am distressed because I cannot face them'. In the one case the emphasis is on introspection, and is relatively independent of the views of others. In the other, what matters is that relationships are jeopardized, and — at the extreme — the subject would feel no distress if his misdeeds were known to no-one but himself. Put in this way, the difference (which is obviously a continuum rather than a clear dichotomy) corresponds to some extent with the difference we have already noted between cultures which are individualistic and introspective as against those in which the self is conceptualized much more in terms of interactions: 'inner-directed' as against 'other-directed'. This is a matter in which it is almost impossible to extricate ourselves from our cultural conditioning. We are almost bound to feel that a person who does something wrong, *but only starts to feel bad about it when he is found out*, is displaying a 'lower' standard of morality. Even if this feeling is inescapable, we can at least try to counteract any moralizing tendency in ourselves by realizing that there is a cultural difference, and some people are brought up to be more other-directed and less inner-directed, so this is not a simple moral issue. A practical consequence is that guilt is not a reliable indicator of depressive illness in every culture, and we should not expect to encounter it everywhere.[6] Nor should we be surprised to find that public shame is a potent cause of emotional crises. In an Asian family in Britain, for example, if one member is behaving unacceptably and this eventually leads to a crisis (perhaps admission to hospital following an overdose), the rest of the family sometimes seem to be mainly distressed by 'What will the neighbours say?' — a consideration that the British practitioner may think contemptible. This is not to say that British families do not worry about 'loss of face' — of course they do — but in Asian cultures it seems to occupy a more central position.

ILLNESS AS SOCIAL DYSFUNCTION

Consider the following scene. The patient, an Asian woman, was discharged from hospital a month ago after successful treatment of a short-term illness. She has returned to the clinic for a follow-up visit, accompanied by her husband.

> *Psychiatrist* (English-speaking): 'How is your wife getting on now?'
> *Husband:* 'She is very well now doctor. She is fine. She is looking after the house. She is cooking the food, she is caring for the baby. Thank you, so much . . .'
> *Psychiatrist:* 'Good. I am glad she is able to do those things: and is she feeling well herself?'

(Brief conversation between husband and wife)

> *Husband:* 'She is very well now, doctor, she is able to look after the family, she is cooking the food, I am able to go back to work now . . .'
> *Psychiatrist:* 'Yes, yes, but please ask her now does she feel in herself? Is she happy, is her mind clear? Is she *feeling* all right?'

(A further lengthy conversation. Husband and wife both evidently perplexed, but wanting to answer the question helpfully.)

> *Husband:* 'She is very happy now, doctor, because she is able to do the cooking, she is able to look after the family, she is able to care for the baby, she is able to clean the house. Thank you very much . . .'

This is not a verbatim account and the conversation has been abbreviated, but the experience is a familiar one to psychiatrists working in Pakistan and among Indians and Pakistanis in Britain. It exemplifies the linguistic problems in introspection which have already been discussed, but the other message which seems to come across is that the important criterion of health is the ability to carry out one's obligations, do one's work, fulfil one's role. If you can do these things you are well, if you are unable to do them you are ill, and no more need be said. Any further probing by the practitioner may be seen as either friendly or impertinent curiosity, but not strictly relevant either way. This criterion of health, albeit somewhat narrow, is not unattractive to the busy practitioner who has grown weary of patients who think that all forms of unhappiness are somehow 'pathological' and should be cured medically.

NOTES

1   This is based on the assumption that there is an entity, 'Depressive Illness', which appears in various cultural disguises (see Appendix 1). Most epidemio-logical studies start from this premise: e.g. Pfeiffer (1968) reviewed published accounts of depression in 22 non-European countries and concluded that the 'core symptoms' were mood change, diurnal variation, loss of appetite, sleep, and libido, and some somatic complaints, whereas guilt, hopelessness, and suicidal tendencies were cultural variables. See also Murphy, Wittkower, and Chance (1964). Some other writers have contested the basic premise. Kleinman, for example, taking a more anthropological viewpoint, rejects the idea of depression (or any mental illness) as:

> 'an entity, a thing to be "discovered" in pure form under the layers of cultural camouflage . . . There can be no stripping away of layers of cultural accretion in order to isolate a culture-free entity. Culture shapes disease, first by shaping our explanations of disease. . . .'   (Kleinman 1977 : 4)

In their classic study of the Yoruba, Leighton and his colleagues noted that:

> 'The symptom-pattern of depression as such — psychotic or psychoneu-rotic — was not volunteered by our informants, and when described to them was not immediately accepted as something familiar.'
>
> (Leighton *et al.* 1963)

They record that many of the symptoms of depression came up in other contexts, as part of various different, culture-specific, symptom-clusters.

   The logic of this argument is that the symptom-clusters (syndromes) found in each culture should be accepted and described *as they are*, not dismantled and rearranged to conform to European typology. This approach has been adopted by some epidemiologists (e.g. Carstairs and Kapur 1976). See also Kessel (1965). Kleinman's appeal for cultural relativism is both cogent and timely, but it makes for problems in intercultural comparisons and it does not immediately help the practitioner who wishes to know how to recognize those 'illnesses' for which he has effective treatments available.

2   G. Mahy, Consultant Psychiatrist, Barbados, and F. Knight, Department of Psychiatry, Kingstown, Jamaica. Personal communications.

3   For examples of this mode of thinking see Carothers (1947, 1951, 1953), Ack-ernecht (1948). The argument has been extended to include black Americans (e.g. Babcock 1954) but when all other variables are controlled it seems likely that black Americans are not particularly prone to somatization (Tonks *et al.* 1970).

4   'Available scientific knowledge provides no basis for believing that the groups of mankind differ in their innate capacity for intellectual and emotional development.'

   'Genetic differences are of little significance in determining the social and cultural differences between groups.'   (UNESCO 1952)

5   There are problems even between closely related languages. It is impossible, for example, to translate 'sense of humour' precisely into French. The German

word '*Angst*' is not the same as the English word 'anxiety' — it describes a mood-state for which no exact English translation exists. These problems can be got round with a suitable periphrasis, but the questions undergo some alteration of form and emphasis, and therefore (perhaps) of meaning. (See, for an example, Murphy, Saunier, and Vachon-Spilka 1968.)

6 Rao noted the relative absence of guilt in Indian depressives and linked it to the Hindu concept of Karma (Rao 1973). Bavington noted that in Pathans (a culture where great importance is attached to family honour), guilt was significantly present in only about one half of depressed patients: it was of mild degree, and he comments that it was difficult to find suitable expressions in colloquial Pushto to identify the experience correctly (Bavington 1981 and personal communication). See also Neki (1973) and Yap (1965). Murphy and his colleagues suggested that Christian teaching fosters a sense of culpability and predisposes to expressions of guilt (Murphy, Wittkower, and Chance 1964, 1967).

11

Cultural Pitfalls
in the Recognition of
Mania

Some authors have suggested that people of Afro-Caribbean descent are liable to a particular form of reaction which is seldom seen elsewhere, and the name 'West Indian Psychosis' has even been coined for it (Tewfik and Okasha 1965). The characteristics of the syndrome are said to be excitement and over-activity, with pressure of thought and speech, sometimes accompanied by cognitive confusion with subsequent loss of memory. Bizarre behaviour may occur (e.g. removal of clothes in public), and violence is common, especially if attempts are made forcibly to restrain the patient. Talk is often fragmented or incoherent, and there often seems to be some paranoid ideation, which stops short of systematized or complex delusions.

In purely descriptive terms, such behaviour may be called *manic*. In our diagnostic classication *mania* is an endogenous psychosis (see Appendix 1) and in British subjects, manic behaviour is almost always a symptom of mania. If Afro-Caribbean subjects are indeed peculiarly prone to manic behaviour, we must ask: is this group particularly prone to the disease, *mania*, or can manic behaviour in this group mean something other than mania? This is an important question, because the diagnosis of mania (as an endogenous psychosis) has implications regarding causation, prognosis, and methods of treatment that are fairly standardized and reasonably effective.

It is quite possible that mania as an endogenous psychosis may occur with different prevalence in different groups. As with the other psychoses, there is some tendency for inheritance, if not of the disorder itself, at least of the propensity to develop it: and this propensity may well be different in different genetic pools. But we do not yet have reliable incidence figures world-wide even for manic-depressive psychosis, (which is one of the most clear-cut of all psychiatric diagnoses), nor do we know what factors cause a preponderance of either manic or depressive episodes in the course of the disorder. Among the indigenous English, depressive episodes greatly outnumber manic ones. It is possible that among Afro-Caribbeans the ratio is reversed for purely genetic reasons. It is also possible that what differs is the *salience*, rather than the *prevalence* of the disorders.

A twenty-three-year-old student was admitted to hospital in a state of wild excitement. He had been born in Jamaica, and came to Britain at the age of thirteen. He has no previous history of psychiatric disorder, nor was there any family history. The story was that a fight had broken out in a public house, and during the disturbance the patient, who was normally a quiet and unassuming person, had 'gone absolutely berserk', and caused a great deal of damage to property until apprehended by the police. In custody he was described as 'like a wild animal' and collected some additional charges for assaulting the police and resisting arrest. On admission to hospital he was noted to be restless and over-active, with continuous garbled speech and constant threats of violence. He made frequent references to 'the power in him', and seemed to have grandiose delusions, demanding instant obedience from the examining doctor and nurses. His condition remained the same for two days, during which despite heavy sedation he did not sleep, he refused food on some occasions and ate voraciously on others, and his constant shouting caused considerable disturbance. On the third day he was quieter and this was attributed to the cumulative effects of large doses of chlor-promazine. He remained somewhat overactive, overtalkative, and grandiose in his behaviour for a further three days and then slowly reverted to his normal modest and polite self. At that stage he was unable to remember the circumstances of his admission, having only fragmentary recollections of a quarrel, and of being angry in police custody. When the full story had been pieced together, it transpired that he was due to take an examination the following week and was worried about it, and two days earlier he had been rejected by his girl friend after a trivial quarrel. He also had a longstanding mild grievance against his landlord which had not been openly expressed. He admitted that he had been 'in low spirits' on the evening in question, and had found the jovial conviviality of his companions irritating.

During the second week in hospital chlorpromazine was slowly withdrawn and he remained quite normal, and was discharged. He was seen as an out-patient for the next seven months, after which he left the area having passed his exams at a deferred sitting. His subsequent career is not known.

This case is not untypical. His disorder looked like acute mania — indeed, as a description of his behaviour there is no other word than manic — but as one got to know him better the importance of the stresses that he was under became more obvious. His behaviour became almost understandable in the light of those stresses; he derived considerable relief from talking about them, and from facing the need to make some practical decisions. The non-psychiatrist reader will not find this history extraordinary and nor will the psychodynamically-orientated clinician who anticipates a psychological rather than a biological explanation for behaviour. Most clinicians recognize that life-stresses can trigger an episode of mania in a predisposed subject, and a recent research paper has drawn fresh attention to this point.[1] But most British clinicians have a tendency to consider mania within a biological rather than a psychological frame of reference. One authority states: 'It would seem questionable from the available data that reactive mania exists at all' (Winokur, Clayton, and Reich 1969 : 30). In non-European cultures the syndrome of 'reactive mania' or 'reactive excitation' is well recognized[2] as a stress reaction.[3]

REACTIVE EXCITATION

Leaving aside semantic arguments, the important point is that when an African, Afro-Caribbean, or Asian patient behaves in a manner that would, in a British patient, point to a diagnosis of mania, the practitioner should keep in mind the possibility that this is a stress reaction, and not an attack of an endogenous psychosis (Littlewood and Lipsedge 1977, 1981). This is, of course, the approach we are accustomed to take to depression. We ask to what entent it is endogenous, to what extent reactive, and we know that to whatever extent stresses, personality features, and external circumstances play a part in causation, to that extent they have to be included in treatment if it is to be successful. The same approach should be applied to states of excitement. This is summarized in *Table 11(1)*. Category 4 in this scheme is one that is likely to catch the British practitioner unawares, and presumably accounts for the 'West Indian Psychosis' designation. That term is not really satisfactory however, because it implies that Afro-Caribbeans are unusual because they may react to stress in this way. It would be more accurate to say that in world terms the British are unusual because they do not.

The stereotype of the 'wild West Indian' presumably owes something to this propensity to reactive excitation. It is an unfortunate stereotype, since West Indians may develop a whole variety of psychiatric conditions and present them with the same repertoire of symptoms as anyone else. Stereotypes, however, have a life of their own, and the image of the big wild, dangerous black man or woman is deeply imprinted in many white

Table 11 (1)

	Depression	*Excitement*
ENDOGENOUS Biological, genetic factors. Stress not primary cause. ↑ ⎮ ⎮ ⎮ ⋁	**1** *'Endogenous depression'* (Psychotic depression). Recognized in all cultures, but symptoms may differ.	**3** *'Mania'* Recognized in all cultures. Less common than depression.
REACTIVE Response to stress, conflict, 'neurotic' rather than 'psychotic'.	**2** *'Reactive depression'* Common in Britain. In other cultures may be regarded as not being a 'medical' problem.	**4** *'Reactive excitation'* ('reactive mania'). Rare among British but well known elsewhere.

people's minds. This may be partly because there are some West Indians (especially Jamaicans) whose manner of speaking is (to English ears) rather sharp, intense, abrupt, and hard-edged, with sudden changes of pitch, coupled with an ebullience of manner that suggests intense emotion or extraversion.[4] Also, there is a great deal of genuine anger, frustration, and bitterness among certain sections of the Afro-Caribbean community in Britain, and it causes acts of violence that attract a great deal of media coverage. Littlewood and Cross (1980) have reported that black patients are more likely than whites to be admitted to hospital under compulsion or with the aid of the police. The syndrome of reactive excitation (and other psychogenic psychoses) may partly explain this, but it is also possible that the stereotype of 'wildness' may provoke those who intervene in crisis situations into an over-reaction that aggravates matters further.[5] The practitioner who is confronted by an angry, emotionally disturbed black person must do what he can to avoid confrontation, and create an atmosphere of acceptance within which communication can occur and under-standing can become possible. This is, of course, exactly what he would do in the case of a white person.

NOTES

1 Ambelas (1979) studied sixty-seven consecutive cases of mania, diagnosed by strict criteria, and found stressful life-events had occurred in the four weeks preceding onset of fourteen cases, which was significantly higher than a control group. Ambelas points out that reactive mania is a concept included in European literature but neglected in Britain, and challenges the prevailing view that mania is never reactive or psychogenic (Ambelas 1979).

2 Admission statistics, Black Rock Mental Hospital, Barbados 1978. The diagnosis 'Reactive excitations' (ICD 298.1) was applied to seventeen female and three male patients (respectively 4.3 per cent and 0.5 per cent of admissions). All were first admissions, and the age groups were:

15-20	21-30	31-40	41-50	51-70	70+
2	6	10	1	0	1

These statistics are subject to the usual vagaries and idiosyncracies of categorization, but they are at least suggestive, and are supported by the clinical experience of psychiatrists in Barbados and Jamaica. (I am indebted to Dr George Mahy for permission to study hospital records and to the Records Officer for assistance in doing so.)

3 There is a problem of nomenclature. If the term 'mania' is reserved for the endogenous psychosis then 'reactive mania' is a nonsense, and the preferred term would be 'reactive excitation' (which is used in the International Classification of Disease). If 'mania' is used purely as a descriptive term without preconceptions as to cause, then reactive mania is a perfectly proper description, and more recognisable. Transcultural studies of mania are rare. (See Leff, Fisher, and Bertebren 1967).

4 The extravert ebullience of Afro-Caribbean people is a racial stereotype which draws support from loud music at late night parties, public carnivals, and back-slapping joviality. Somehow the image of Caribbean islanders as good-natured, easy going and indolent people who take nothing seriously except cricket, co-exists with the image of violent angry aggressiveness and criminality in Britain: but stereotypes do not have to be logical. In a study of school children, Hill found no significant difference between those of English and those of West Indian parents on the Extraversion score of the Eysenck Junior Personality Inventory (Hill 1975).

5 There is evidence that Afro-Caribbean patients are more likely to be admitted to hospital unwillingly or with the aid of police (Rwegellera 1980; Kelleher and Copeland 1972). Studies in Leicester and Bradford suggest that this finding does not apply to Asian patients (Hitch and Clegg 1980; Joseph 1978; Shaikh and Bhate 1980).

Cultural Pitfalls
in the Recognition of
Schizophrenia

Schizophrenia is a severely disabling mental illness (see Appendix 1) which apparently exists throughout the world. Psychiatrists working in many different ethnic and cultural groups are in substantial agreement about its 'core symptoms' (WHO 1972). It is important to diagnose the disorder when it is present, because effective treatment is possible, but it is equally important not to diagnose it when it is not present, because in the present state of knowledge and attitudes, a diagnosis of schizophrenia is a statement with far-reaching consequences for the person concerned. Not only psychiatrists, but people in general, are apt to react differently to patients to whom this label has been attached.

Our diagnostic confusion is twofold. First, there is no general agreement about the boundaries of the category. If we drew up a list of eight features that are common in schizophrenia and not in other conditions, we would have no diagnostic problem in a case in which all eight features were present.[1] But such a case would be rare: usually we would accept the diagnosis on the strength of five or six features. But what if only three are present? Two psychiatrists might then disagree — not necessarily about the symptoms, their supposed causes, the appropriate treatment, or the expected prognosis, but simply on the semantic issue of whether or not such a case falls within the boundaries of the term 'schizophrenia' in the sense in which they have each become accustomed to using that term. This is particularly likely to happen between psychiatrists from different countries with different academic traditions.

In Britain, but not in Europe or America, the term schizophrenia is often used with an unstated implication of 'biological' factors of causation. There is assumed to be a latent abnormality that may be activated by, but is not entirely caused by, environmental or psychological factors. Therefore when breakdown appears to be a simple and direct consequence of stress, even if the symptoms are to some extent 'schizophrenic' in type, the patient will not be regarded as 'a schizo-phrenic' if the clinician believes that he can understand the psychological causes. *To whatever extent the clinician perceives psychodynamic or exogenous factors to be relevant to the mental breakdown, to that extent he is likely to veer away from the diagnosis 'schizophrenia' in favour of some other diagnostic category.* Accepting this convention, we can use the word 'schizophreniform' for symptoms that are found in schizophrenia and usually point in the direction of that diagnosis. Our second cause of confusion is that some schizophreniform symptoms may be explicable psychologically in one culture but not in another. When all or even most of the classic signs of schizophrenia are present we shall have no diagnostic problem; but in respect of individual symptoms — delusions, hallucinations, thought disorder, paranoia, and so on — we have to ask, to what else might they be due, other than schizophrenia?

DELUSIONS

A delusion is a false belief, but it is not evidence of mental illness unless it is not only false but out of keeping with the subject's normal beliefs. Thus a British scientist who announced that he was a victim of Voodoo would be a fit subject for psychiatric examination, whereas a Haitian farmer would not. The question is not how odd does he seem to *you* (a British middle-class practitioner), but how odd does he seem to *his fellows*. This demands a knowledge of the belief-systems of the particular culture which the practitioner may not possess, but he should not jump to conclusions until he has checked with someone who does have that knowledge. This is the first pitfall and is obvious. The second is the opposite: to assume that a belief is culturally normal when it is, in fact, abnormal. This pitfall lies in wait for the practitioner who has developed some degree of cultural sensitivity. We must not forget that whenever a person develops a psychotic delusion, it will be manufactured from, and expressed in terms of, the prevailing culture. Thus a paranoid patient in Britian may complain that television cameras are following him about, whereas a Pathan may say that a magic evil object has been secretly introduced into his house. The second statement is not necessarily any more 'normal' than the first.[2]

LINGUISTIC MISUNDERSTANDINGS

Mistakes can occur through simple linguistic misunderstandings. A British general practitioner received a letter from one of his Pakistani patients, a newly married man. The letter was written in English and included the statement that following sexual intercourse with his wife 'everytime a lot of money comes out of her hole'. The GP wrote to the local psychiatrist stating: 'He handed me this extraordinary letter. When he talks of money coming out of his wife's vagina, one wonders if he is delusional . . . and not merely suffering from a psychoneurosis . . .'. Fortunately the psychiatrist understood Urdu, and realized that the Urdu word *money* (or *Muni*) is the Urdu word for semen! He had noticed post-coital leakage and was worried lest his wife fail to become pregnant.[3] Curious effects may arise when an idiomatic usage is imperfectly understood as with the man who was 'hunting the wild geese' in a hospital corridor.[4] Just as English has taken in several Hindi words (e.g. Pukha, Sahib) so Indians use several English words and phrases. In Bengali the term 'Royal Family' can be used to denote 'posh' or 'respectable'. Thus it happened that when a Bengali man was picked up by the police in the centre of Bradford, the police surgeon could not get much out of him because of his poor English, but he did seem to keep on expressing this grandiose delusion about being related to royalty.

The patois of some Caribbean islanders provides scope for misunderstandings, especially when it is combined with a fundamentalist religious faith. Statements like 'The good Lord is speaking to me' should not be accepted at face value. The Rastafari usage of 'I-and-' sounds very odd when first heard, and a statement such as 'I-and-I walking down the street' might suggest some kind of thought disorder.

SUPERSTITION AND MAGICAL BELIEFS

We have stressed that many immigrants from rural communities have beliefs and attitudes characteristic of peasants (see Chapter 4). They believe that it is possible for one human being to influence the health or well-being of another by action at a distance, without the mechanism by which the influence is transmitted being apparent, and that some people are particularly skilful at doing this and regularly exercise their powers against people whom they dislike or for payment. The majority of mankind subscribe to such beliefs, including many indigenous British people, though they may not admit it openly. In the West Indies the Obeah man (or woman) is a powerful figure. A sufferer may say that his enemy has 'put an Obeah on him', and employ his own Obeah man for protection and retaliation. Asian patients may be observed wearing '*Tavees*', which are protective charms hung round the neck. Orthodox religion is used as a defence against witchcraft, so verses from the Koran may be used as *Tavees*. Sometimes a thread is tied round a limb or a digit as a protective amulet. (If this is discovered in the course of a medical examination it should be left undisturbed. There are cases on record of a nurse insisting on the removal of such a thread when preparing a patient for operation — little realizing that it had been obtained specially to protect against the perils of the operation!)

Severe mental illness, with its distressing and mystifying qualities, is an obvious subject for magical or supernatural explanations. Kiev notes that:

> 'in most pre-technical, pre-literate, and underdeveloped cultures (mental illness) has invariably been explained by supernatural concepts of taboo violation, witchcraft, the intrusion of harmful objects into the body, or loss of a vital substance from the body and possession by angry or evil spirits . . .'   (Kiev 1972 : 103)

If insanity is inflicted by Gods or ancestral spirits this is attributed to violation of taboos or other misbehaviour, in which case the affliction is in some sense the sufferer's own fault. Witchcraft, however, may cause quite undeserved insanity. It is often accomplished by surreptitious administration of harmful substances which upset the body's natural equilibrium. Hence, accusations of poisoning and accusations of witchcraft are not mutually exclusive: they often go together.

Magical explanations of illness are a favourite subject for anthropological research, but for the practitioner their diagnostic significance is slight. They do not indicate either the presence or absence of schizophrenia.

A Sikh woman living in Bradford jumped out of a first-floor window and sustained multiple fractures. She stated that this was the result of a curse. She had recently made a visit to India, and while there had started to feel ill. She had quarrelled with a relative and assumed that her symptoms were the result of witchcraft. When the symptoms continued after her return to Britain she became really worried. She consulted a local *Davi* (religious healer) who confirmed her fears, and provided her with magic talismans (*Tavees*) to wear on her body for protection. This produced transient reassurance, but her husband was unimpressed and insisted that she remove the *Tavees*. When she did so, she panicked and jumped out of the window. The presentation — impulsive irrational behaviour in association with paranoid delusions — was suggestive of schizophrenia, but when the cultural 'red herrings' were disregarded, her illness proved to be a simple depressive illness and responded completely to antidepressant treatment.

This was an example of a 'delusion' which turned out to be a culturally valid belief. Sometimes, however, it works the other way. A young high-caste Hindu Brahmin became withdrawn and abstracted, uttered incomprehensible fragmented speech, and alternated between inert passivity and violent purposeless activity including rolling on the ground. His family were unable to control him and brought him to the psychiatric unit to be cared for. But, they said, they did not want him to have any treatment, since his behaviour was not due to illness but showed that he was passing through a particular and important phase in his spiritual development, from which he would shortly emerge with benefit. The family's wishes were respected for three weeks, during which he deteriorated further until eventually by mutual agreement treatment was commenced. The diagnosis of schizophrenia has been confirmed by subsequent developments.

Superstitious beliefs are by no means confined to the so-called Third World. Similar diagnostic problems are encountered by clinicians in European industrial centres who have migrant-worker patients from rural areas of southern Europe.[5]

POSSESSION STATES

'Possession' refers to a take-over of the subject's will, in fact usually his whole mind and body, by some external force or spirit. The force is usually envisaged as a supernatural being, either a god or a ghost. As long as he is possessed, the subject is held to be not responsible for his actions — they are not 'his' actions at all, but the actions of the spirit which controls him. The term 'possessed' is used in two slightly different ways.

Ritual possession

This is an acute and short-lived state of dissociation produced deliberately as part of a ceremony devised for the purpose. Sargant (1973) has collected examples of ritual possession from various parts of the world, and his comprehensive review of the subject as seen through the eyes of the psychiatrist is so well-known that it requires only a brief precis here. A possession ceremony usually involves prolonged dancing to very loud and rhythmic music in a setting of heightened group emotion. There is a charismatic leader who is credited with supernatural powers and he or she sets out quite deliberately to generate intense excitement in the participants, frequently using macabre, gruesome, or sexual elements to break down inhibitions and create the expectation that something extraordinary and highly significant is about to happen. The participants in this physically and emotionally strenuous activity share this expectation and sooner or later one of them goes into the state of possession. This is often heralded by some sort of convulsion, after which the possessed subject exhibits the behaviour characteristic of the spirit by which he is now taken over. He may, for example, wriggle like a snake, cheep like a bird, or display astonishing gymnastic ability. His actions and utterances while in this state are accorded great significance, since he is now regarded as a direct channel to the supernatural world. His state of possession usually terminates in collapse, from which he is slowly brought back to full consciousness by his friends. Hypnosis plays a part in the induction of possession, and drugs may also be used. As with other hypnotic and dissociated states, some people are more easily affected than others, and repetition makes the transition easier. Some regular participants can become possessed quite easily whenever they are given the right stimuli, and can be induced to display abnormal behaviour such as fire-walking and fire-eating as a matter of routine, even as a tourist attraction.[6]

Sargent has drawn interesting comparisons between possession ceremonies in Voodoo and other animistic religions, the behaviour of young devotees at pop concerts and discotheques, the hysterical states sometimes seen in acute battle neuroses (and their treatment by abreaction), and the techniques of religious conversion employed by some Christian evangelists. The comparisons are persuasive. He describes the mechanism of dissociation in terms of Pavlovian psychology, but alternative explanations are possible (see also Lewis 1971).

States of altered consciousness, self-induced or induced by group excitement or overwhelming emotion are not, therefore, the prerogative of any one culture, and although the induction techniques vary according to culture they have basic similarities. The term 'possession' will be used by people whose religious beliefs include spirits – holy or unholy – which are available for intervention in human affairs. Others will describe the experience in other terms.

'Possession' as ascribed aetiology

The other sense in which the word 'possessed' may be used by a patient or a patient's relative is as an explanation for mental disorder of a less acute and dramatic kind, in fact any kind of mental aberration for which no other explanation is apparent. This is in no way diagnostic. It may be applied to hysteria, anxiety, phobic and other neurotic states, psychosis, or physical illness. It is perplexing for any individual to find himself gripped by feelings of panic for no obvious reason, or to feel compelled to carry out actions that he knows are at variance with his conscious wishes. If the subject's belief-systems can accommodate a supernatural explanation it may be used. In schizophrenia the hallucinations, passivity feelings, and ideas of influence lend themselves to this kind of interpretation.

HALLUCINATIONS

Hallucinations, which in British patients commonly point towards a diagnosis of either schizophrenia or some organic condition, do not necessarily have the same meaning elsewhere. For example, among Asian women, and especially teenage girls, the commonest cause of hallucinations is not schizophrenia but hysteria. Some reaons for this are discussed in the section on hysteria.

SCHIZOPHRENIC THOUGHT DISORDER

As well as thinking abnormal thoughts (e.g. delusions) the schizophrenic patient often puts his thoughts together in an abnormal manner. The *thought process* is affected as well as the *thought content*. (The prefix 'Schiz-' which means 'splitting', refers to this fragmentation of thinking, not, as laymen suppose, to a 'split personality' on the Jekyll and Hyde model.) When typically schizophrenic thought *process* disorder can be detected it has great diagnostic significance because it is relatively specific. It is a particularly useful sign to elicit in patients from unfamiliar cultures, because in those patients other signs (delusions, hallucinations, excitement, incongruity) may be unreliable.

Unfortunately, while this abnormality is probably universal, it is of all psychiatric abnormalities the most dependent on language. Unless the patient and the diagnostician have a common language, in which both are really fluent, it is quite impossible to be sure whether the hesitations and discontinuities are linguistic or psychotic. This is one of the points at which it may be helpful to utilize the services of an interpreter. Not that the interpreter will be able to translate the thought-disordered speech: on the contrary, he will find it quite impossible to do so, since the words are put together in an idiosyncratic fashion that cannot be reproduced. Thought disorder is elicited at second hand by asking the interpreter to describe *why* he is unable to reproduce it.

PSYCHOGENIC PSYCHOSIS: THE ACUTE
SCHIZOPHRENIFORM STRESS REACTION

Suppose that an English patient is admitted to a psychiatric hospital displaying paranoid delusions accompanied by hallucinations, fragmentation of thought, incongruity of mood, and bizarre unpredictable behaviour, all of which have developed acutely during the preceding days or weeks. He or she is almost certain to receive a diagnosis of schizophrenia. Suppose that the patient's friends or relatives explain that this has all happened because of some recent trauma or disaster, or emotional conflict. Their views will be noted, but the clinician will probably have a private conviction that the events they describe were nothing more than trigger factors. He will probably assume that the patient had a 'schizophrenic predispositon' and would be at risk for developing the illness sooner or later, with or without a precipitating stress. English patients under stress may develop anxiety, depression, hysterical disabilities and many other things, but the classical schizophreniform manifestations — Schneider's 'First Rank Symptoms' — are not usually prominent in the repertoire of stress responses.

This generalization does not hold good outside Europe. In Asia, Africa, the Caribbean, and probably elsewhere, schizophreniform symptoms may be produced purely as a stress reaction, and such a reaction does not necessarily indicate a schizophrenic predisposition. It follows that when we are dealing with an Asian or Afro-Caribbean subject who appears to be suffering from acute schizophrenia, we should pay full attention to psychological and environmental factors. The conflicts and traumas mentioned by the relatives may be genuine causes, not merely trigger factors. It may be wrong to assume that the illness would have developed sooner or later.

At the time of onset, the symptoms of psychogenic psychosis may be quite indistinguishable from acute schizophrenia, though some points of difference have been listed by continental European writers, for example, Faergeman (1963). According to Faergeman, hallucinations are less common in the psychogenic form, but in our own experience of Asian and Afro-Caribbean patients this is not a reliable discriminator, and indeed we have the impression that visual hallucinations, and hallucinations of more than one modality at a time, are pointers towards a psychogenic aetiology, as also are cognitive confusion, including misperception and disorientation. Another important clue is prompt spontaneous recovery. It is not uncommon to admit someone to hospital one day, give them a single dose of a sedative phenothiazine and find them totally recovered in the morning, with amnesia for the previous day's events. This initial recovery is not necessarily permanent.

Treatment may have to include phenothiazine drugs in the acute phase, but as with other reactive conditions drugs alone do not solve the problem, and it is essential to understand the underlying stresses and help the patient to do something about them. Whereas most schizophrenics are advised to continue taking medication for a long period after recovery, this is not necessary in these patients, and merely confuses the issue — and the patient.

Referring back to the chart we constructed to accomodate Reactive Excitation (Chapter 11 *Table 11(1)* we may now add two more boxes and produce *Table 12(1)*. It is particularly important that patients with

Table 12 (1)

	Depression	Excitement	Schiz . . .
ENDOGENOUS Biological, genetic factors. Stress not primary cause. ↑ | | | | ↓	1 'Endogenous depression' (psychotic depression). Recognized in all cultures, but symptoms may differ.	3 'Mania' Recognized in all cultures. Less common than depression.	5 'Schizophrenia' Probably exists everywhere.
REACTIVE Response to stress, conflict, 'Neurotic' rather than 'psychotic'.	2 'Reactive depression' Common in Britain. In other cultures may be regarded as not being a 'medical' problem.	4 'Reactive excitation' ('reactive mania'). Rare among British but well known elsewhere. Psychogenic psychoses.	6 'Acute Schizophreniform stress reaction'

psychogenic psychoses are not labelled schizophrenic, as this diagnosis distorts the attitude which other people will take towards the patient for years to come.

CANNABIS

Cannabis intoxication may produce an acute confusional state with hallucinations, paranoia, and excitement resembling an acute schizophreniform reaction. The condition usually clears up spontaneously but may take several days to do so, and admission to hospital may be required. The differentation from acute schizophrenia or other toxic confusional states is usually made retrospectively when the history of cannabis-taking has been obtained. Cannabis is readily available in the northern parts of the Indian subcontinent and throughout the Caribbean, and its use is not confined to any particular age-group or section of the population. Cannabis is known as *Ganja* in the Caribbean, and in the Indian subcontinent it is called *Charras* when smoked, or

Bhang if taken as a drink. Chronic use is said to produce a state of indolent withdrawal not unlike chronic schizophrenia.

NOTES

1 See e.g. Schneider's list of 'first-rank' symptoms of schizophrenia (Schneider 1959). A valuable review article is Kendall (1972).

2 Chandrasena summarizes this as follows: cultural beliefs can (a) be mistaken for mental illness or (b) conceal the existence of mental illness; (c) when mental illness is present, the cultural beliefs and the delusional beliefs must be distinguished (Chandrasena 1979). Many Indian and Pakistani authors have pointed out that the contents of delusions in Asian schizophrenics are different from those commonly found in Europe. They tend to have religious, super-stitious, and sexual components especially (see for example Ahmed 1978 or Kiev 1963).

3 I am indebted to Dr Sheikh, Consultant Psychiatrist, Worcester for sending me this (true) illustrative example.

4 He was, of course, indignant because he had been sent on a wild goose chase. The story is probably apocryphal.

5 The experience of Swiss psychiatrists dealing with migrant patients from south Italy is strikingly similar to the experience of British psychiatrists with Pakistani patients. This need not surprise us, since both sets of patients have come from peasant cultures (see Chapter 4). For example, see Risso and Böker (1974). (Summarized in Zwingmann (1977).)

6 Author's observation. Port-au-Prince, Haiti, 1979.

Cultural Pitfalls
in the Recognition of
Paranoia

For present purposes 'paranoia' means feelings of persecution. A person is described as paranoid if he believes he is being persecuted, threatened, victimized, discriminated against, reviled, hated, jeered at or joked about, plotted against, or otherwise maltreated; if he believes this treatment to be unjust and undeserved; and if there is no objective evidence of the truth of his assertions. A person who habitually confronts life with a cautious, untrusting attitude, suspiciously seeking the hidden catch in every proposition, may be called a *paranoid personality*. A person who claimed that an electronic device had been secretly implanted in his head, whereby his every thought was being monitored by agents of a foreign power, would be said to be suffering from a paranoid delusion (and such a delusion would be suggestive, though by no means conclusive, evidence of schizophrenia).

PARANOIA AND OPPRESSION

Among the causes of stress listed in Part II, we have included the effects of belonging to a minority group, particularly if the minority is subjected to discrimination or oppression. Few will dispute that ethnic minorities in Britain are at a disadvantage in respect of housing, education, employment, social status, and so on. What, then, are we to make of the patient or client who says he is being persecuted? Is this to be regarded as paranoia?

To some people the answer to this seems obvious. There are spokesmen in the ethnic minorities who state that persecution by the rest of society is the most important single fact of life for their people (especially if they are black). This is neatly expressed by one writer: 'Adapting from one culture to another can be compared to learning to eat with your left hand when you have been trained to eat with your right hand. But for ethnic minorities, adapting to a racist culture is like learning not to eat at all' (Dharamsi 1976). Many white people who are aware of what really goes on, and are committed to the cause of race relations, would agree with that. To such people, all the other factors considered so far will appear trivial by comparison.

The points that have already been made on this subject (see Chapter 6) need not be repeated here, though they must never be overlooked. For present purposes, however, there are two propositions to be considered:

(1) Oppression makes people paranoid.
(2) A person who complains about oppression is in danger of being labelled as paranoid.

Either or both of these propositions may be true, and common sense would support both. But to the extent that the second is true it must cast doubt on anything that is said about the first.

One way of approaching this is to ask whether psychiatric patients who are from minority groups are more paranoid, or include paranoia among their symptoms, more often than other psychiatric patients. Several studies have shown that they do (Prange 1959; Mezey 1960a, 1960b; Kiev 1964; Gordon 1965; Tewfik and Okasha 1965; Carpenter and Brockington 1980; Cochrane 1977) and the term 'alien's paranoid reaction' has been coined (Kino 1951). But it is not easy to decide whether the paranoia is a reaction to the hostility of the host community, or to stresses associated with migration. The author's own experience is somewhat contradictory. We have found one particular group of immigrants who have a high incidence of paranoia: the Poles (Hitch and Rack 1980). The other groups that we have studied (e.g. Pakistanis) do not. It would be wrong to draw nay firm conclusions from this, but it is noteworthy that Pakistanis are more discriminated against and victimized than Poles, so if paranoia were a simple response to persecution one would expect the difference between the two groups to be the other way round.

Another approach is to ask how often patients mention victimization as a cause of their problems. The author's own experience is that Asians and Afro-Caribbeans do so less often than would be expected. In fact, they do not mention discrimination and social inequalities when it would be quite reasonable to do so. This may be because the author is perceived to be a member of the 'establishment', who would not be expected to listen to such complaints; it may be that different responses are obtained when the practitioner is himself a member of the same minority group as the client.

All the same, we might expect that if racism is a major preoccupation it would show up in the content of the paranoid delusions of psychotic patients. Our own impressions do not suggest this. Paranoid delusions in Asian patients include accusations about family members, magic, and witchcraft, more often than persecution by the police, the Government, white employers, or the National Front. If a Pakistani patient states that neighbours are talking about him, they are more often Pakistani neighbours than English ones. If someone is trying to poison him it is more likely to be a wicked uncle than a white workmate, and the ascribed motive is more likely to be an inheritance dispute than racial hostility.[1] By contrast, patients of Eastern European origin include in their delusions the police, television programmes, English workmates, neighbours, and other representatives of the majority 'establishment' (not infrequently including the practitioner himself, who may be accused of poisoning them with the wrong treatment). It is, of course, possible that the Asian or Afro-Caribbean patient who is paranoid against English doctors is a patient that the English doctor never sees.

A third possible approach is a detailed analysis of psychopathology in individual cases, aiming to get beyond the presenting symptoms to the underlying conflicts and tensions. Some such studies have been undertaken but inevitably, only small samples can be studied in this way, and generalizations from such samples are dangerous. The classic 'Psychological Study of the American Negro' by Kardiner and Ovesey (1951) was of this kind. In their twenty-five subjects low self-esteem was a very common feature, and this often led to self-contempt and contempt for blackness. Whites therefore became idealized, and the subject wished to join white society. Being unable to do so made him angry, but because whites were idealized his anger could not be directed against them and was displaced instead on to himself and his fellow blacks. Frustration and impotent anger, frequently repressed or displaced, are the features common to most studies of this kind, and it is not difficult to see how such feelings might eventually produce aggressive or paranoid outbursts. The term 'Black Rage' has become popular recently in this connection. Weinreich has produced studies of black teenagers in Britain; his findings, while they do not contradict this general impression, suggest that the psychopathology is somewhat more complex than this simple model suggests (Weinreich 1979). An Indian or Pakistani in Britain cannot alter his skin, but one thing that he can alter is his religion, and we have come to recognize that a desire to join a Christian church may sometimes be an indicator of low self-esteem.

To the question: 'Does oppression make people paranoid?', therefore, we have no definitive answer. It seems likely that it makes people fearful and angry, and causes problems of identification and self-image; we might anticipate that this would show up in terms of paranoia, but in Britain at the present time we do not have data on which to base such a generalization, probably because there are so many variables that simple cause-and-effect hypotheses are untestable.

The second proposition — that people may be considered paranoid when they express legitimate grievances — can be dealt with more straightforwardly. At one level — admittedly a fairly trivial one — we may observe it happening every day when a misunderstanding arises in an exchange between a member of an ethnic minority and an authority figure. If (for example) a coloured person makes a request and the request is refused, and the reasons for the refusal are not understood, it is very easy for the applicant to assume that the request would have been granted had he been white. His assumption may be correct, or it may not be. Either way, if he says anything about it he may be labelled paranoid. At this level we are not describing a personality-variable, but a communication failure. For the white practitioner who becomes entangled in this kind of situation, the best response is probably as follows:

(1) Check that one has correctly understood the request.
(2) Ask oneself why it is impossible to grant the request: is there any element of choice or not? If there is *any* element of choice, would it be exercized differently *in any way* for a different applicant? If so, has the difference got anything *at all* to do with the applicant's ethnicity? If these questions are faced with complete honesty and the answers are 'No', then it is possible to proceed with a degree of detachment.
(3) Ask oneself why the refusal is not being accepted. What is the applicant's view of the situation? There may be some factor that is so blindingly obvious to the practitioner that he takes it for granted, but of which the applicant is quite unaware. What assumptions is the applicant making, and what may have been his previous experience that would lead him to make those assumptions?

By proceeding along these lines there is at least a chance that misunderstandings will be cleared up, and the applicant will not feel victimized, though he may still be disappointed.

What kind of assumptions might the applicant be making?

(1) That the practitioner is racially prejudiced. This may seem insulting, but since the assumption is presumably based on the applicant's previous experiences with other people, not with him, there is no need for the practitioner to take it personally.
(2) That the practitioner possesses more power or discretion than he actually does. In India and Pakistan, and to a lesser extent in parts of the Caribbean, a person who holds an official government

position has influence beyond the strict limits of the job. He is 'one of them', an establishment figure with influence over other establishment figures and access to unimaginable resources and sanctions. He holds the key to doors that the ordinary man can never open, however just his cause. He can do favours if he wants to. If he refuses, it is because he chooses to refuse, and it is therefore quite reasonable to plead with him instead of taking no for an answer at the first time of asking. Against this background, the Asian who asks his doctor or social worker to use his influence with the Home Office in an immigration appeal may find it difficult to understand that the practitioner has no such influence, and may interpret refusal as a personal rebuff.

(3) That the practitioner is motivated by self-interest, and will not make a move unless there is something in it for him. This seems cynical, but we must realize that in many of the immigrants' countries of origin the social climate is harsh, fending for oneself is a basic rule, and the salaries of many officials are set at low levels on the tacit assumption that they will make a certain amount on the side. Our client may well have met this attitude in officials in his own country, and in his dealings with fellow-countrymen in Britain. He may also have met it among the British, starting with an airport taxi-driver (and not excluding doctors: professional altruism is a sweet dream of the welfare state, but it does not always penetrate the murkier levels of inner-city deprivation).

No doubt many other assumptions could be added to this list. What has all this got to do with paranoia and the diagnosis of schizophrenia? quite a lot. Paranoia, after all, is in the eye of the beholder, so the patient who adopts a suspicious, disbelieving, accusatory attitude to the practitioner is inviting that label. Only when we can understand the assumptions that he is bringing into the relationship, and perceive some possible reasons for those assumptions, are we able to place his paranoia in perspective, deal with it calmly, and not exaggerate its diagnostic importance. Having said that, there are some members of ethnic minorities whose instant explanation for every adversity is in terms of racial prejudice. Failure to get promotion, or pass an exam, or obtain the treatment they desire, or gain as much sympathy as they feel they deserve, is automatically attributed by them to the fact that they are black, or foreigners, or both. Since racial prejudice is endemic in Britain, such people are certain to meet with genuine discrimination sufficiently often to maintain them in their beliefs. Unfortunately, their stereotype of the white racist prevents them, as do all stereotypes, from approaching new situations with an open mind. This attitude can be described as paranoid, but it is a paranoia that has nothing to do with psychosis. It serves a purpose for the individual, which is, 'It's not my fault!'. Many immigrants are unsuccessful, unpopular, and unhappy. To place the blame on other people is a well known psychological defence, and to attribute it to something over which one has no control whatsoever, such as skin colour, relieves one of all responsibility.

Some coloured people who do not seem to be paranoid in their habitual attitudes, nonetheless surprise their white friends from time to time by appearing to over-react on some trivial issue. Why, the white practitioner might ask, should anyone get upset about a gollywog? It is nothing but a cuddly child's toy, a traditional item of nursery equipment which generations of kids have loved and hugged with never a thought of racism in their heads. Surely there is some over-sensitivity here? As usual, we should not start to tell people how they *should* react until we have made the effort to understand why they *do* react. To a white parent, a gollywog is just another soft doll which happens to be black. To many a black parent, its exaggerated racial features and vacuous fixed grin symbolize the white man's patronizing attitude to his 'racial inferiors' through the ages, and all the pejorative overtones of the term 'Wog'.

At this point, it is not uncommon for the black man to say to his white friend: 'Look, you just can't understand. You may be a nice guy, you may be genuinely unprejudiced, you may want to help — but you can't. There's no way a white man can ever know what it's like to live inside a black skin. There's no way you can ever feel the way we feel. You might as well give up — there's just no way in for you'.[2] To a practitioner, and particularly to a psychiatrist, such a statement must be unacceptable. The ability to see the world through another person's eyes is part of his stock-in-trade, one of the things he has been trained in. He may never know what it feels like to be a woman, or a homosexual, or a peasant, or a millionaire, and he will probably never know what it is like to be a refugee or a psychiatric patient, but he does not feel disqualified from trying to understand all those people, even though the understanding can never be complete. To say that skin colour is a greater difference than any of those, an arbitrary and absolute block of a different order, is surely to perpetuate a dangerous myth.

PARANOIA ABOUT THE PAST

What are we to make of the coloured person, usually African or West Indian, who is apparently unable to carry on any conversation without introducing emotional references to the exploitation of their homeland by colonialism? Who, in amongst his current symptoms or problems, intersperses references to slavery and white supremacy? Our customary English patient is unlikely to refer to the Tolpuddle Martyrs or the Enclosures Acts. If he did, this *might* indicate a high degree of political and historical awareness, but unless he is a student of politics or sociology we do not expect him to make such associations in the course of a clinical conversation — and we may begin to suspect him of paranoia or over-inclusive thinking.

With immigrants from former colonial territories we must not jump to such conclusions. There is a sense in which all black people are best treated as students of politics. For one thing, in countries that are relatively small and are experiencing rapid social change, politics have an immediacy that they lack in Britain. The issues about which elections are fought in newly independent states are usually stark, critical, and exciting, and there is a high level of political awareness that is not limited to a committed intelligentsia. In that situation, the stance of the British intellectual who genuinely 'is not interested in politics' is neither appropriate or understandable.

Moreover, many of the New Commonwealth immigrants now in Britain have experienced the processes of political independence in their lifetimes. The trappings of imperial rule were part of the childhood experience of many West Indians now in Britain, and even now not all Caribbean islands have acquired full political autonomy. The British practitioner has probably forgotten how tenacious and how *recent* was Britain's involvement in its colonial territories, and he does not make a connection in his mind between current racial disadvantage, colonial rule, and slavery, but to many Africans or West Indians these are an obvious continuum of degradation (Fanon 1961; Memmi 1957; Mazrui 1979).

It is true that slavery was abolished in the Caribbean almost 150 years ago, but in most of the islands the feudal autocracy of the plantation owners was maintained right up to and within present lifetimes. As recently as 1961 Dr Eric Williams (who became Prime Minister of Trinidad and Tobago) campaigned under the slogan '*Massa Day Done*'. It was time, he proclaimed, to topple the power throughout the world of *Massa* and *Sahib* and *Baas*. Williams's sparkling polemic is instructive reading for anyone interested in Anglo-West Indian relations, because it belongs to the same era as the mass migrations to Britain. The following extracts give a little of the flavour:

'On his West Indian sugar plantations Massa employed unfree labour. He began with the labour of slaves from Africa and followed this with the labour of contract workers from Portugal and China and then from India. . . . To his slave workers from Africa the symbol of

Massa's power was the whip, liberally applied. . . . To his contract workers from India the symbol of Massa's power was the jail.'

'When slavery was abolished in 1833, and Massa was afraid that the emancipated slaves would no longer accept the drudgery and exploit-ation of the slave plantation but would work for themselves on small plots, Massa . . . destroyed the gardens and food plots which the slaves were permitted . . . to force them out of the threat of starvation, to accept starvation wages on the plantation. . . .'

'one such Massa . . . arrived in Nevis about 1680 with ten pounds, a quart of wine, and a Bible. He developed into a big shot, became a planter, merchant, and legislator, and when things turned sour in the nineteenth century he . . . went back to live in the old county of Dorset in England from which his ancestors had migrated to the West Indies . . . Massa left behind Nevis as under-developed as he had found it.'

'Massa's long economic domination . . . reduced the population of the West Indies, whether slave, contract, or free, to the drudgery of the simplest and most unedifying operations, almost unfitting them totally for any intelligent agricultural activity, and giving them a profound and almost permanent distaste for agricultural endeavours.'

'He stated unambiguously (in 1925) that the less education of the children of plantation workers the better . . .'

'there was no civilised society on earth so entirely destitute of learned leisure, literacy and scientific intercourse and liberal recreations.'
(Williams 1973 : 6, 9, 11)

An impassioned election manifesto is not a scientific document, and we need not accept all these statements unreservedly. The point is that this kind of rhetoric, and the conspicuous selfishness and decadence of some estate owners, are still part of the political landscape in the Caribbean, and were part of the life experience of many West Indians now in Britain. The British practitioner may find it irritating to be identified with the plantocracy — with *Massa* — but if the West Indian patient or client makes such an identification, however incongruous, it is not evidence of psychosis. To establish rapport with such a patient a white therapist may have to spend time exploring these attitudes.

LOSS OF CULTURAL CONTINUITY

In the slave trade at least 10 million people were forcibly transported across the Atlantic, and some West Indians and black Americans see this as a racial outrage which its perpetrators must not be allowed to forget. The negro in the Americas is presented as a kind of Flying Dutchman, permanently cut off from the African roots which alone could give him a sense of racial identity and cultural pride. He has been de-cultured and brainwashed. This feeling is expressed by many black writers, castigating:

> 'those British imperialists who in drawing up our educational sylla-
> buses refused to include any mention of great black West Indians
> like Toussaint L'Ouverture, Marcus Garvey, Sylvester Williams. . . .
> We were never told of these men, so that in our search for heroes as
> youngsters we found our men in imperialists like William the
> Conqueror, Benjamin Disraeli and Winston Churchill . . . we were
> never told of the true history of our land whence we were brought –
> Black Africa our fatherland. We were never told that Black Africa
> was more civilised than Europe throughout history . . . we were
> never told that it was as a result of contact with Europeans that the
> glorious path of African development was altered . . . we were never
> told that centuries before the Europeans discovered the world was
> round our fathers made their pilgrimage to Mecca crossing the Sahara
> desert from the ancient empires of Ghana, Mali and Songhai . . . we
> were never told of the black kings and queens whose armies defeated
> early European attempts to capture us.
>
> But instead, to facilitate and prolong our subservience and oppres-
> sion, to this day we were told that we were cannibals and savages.'
>
> (Morris 1966 : 277–78)

As with Massa and the feudalism of the plantations, the British practitioner may feel that all this has nothing to do with him. After all (he
may wish to retort) it was not I who did those things, and it was not
even my ancestors: my ancestors were workers who were exploited by
the prevailing system just as yours were. This response ignores the feeling
of continuity of oppression. We may be able to dissociate ourselves
from the past, but *people who still feel themselves to be oppressed tend
to have long memories.* (Witness, among many possible examples, the
Irish.) If this is 'paranoia' it has nothing to do with mental illness –
except as a diagnostic pitfall.

In practice, debates about historical guilt usually become inconclusive
and sterile; but even if we leave out the question of guilt, the 'rootless-
ness' question requires a little more consideration. It seems to be a
common human attribute to derive pleasure and security from contemplating the historical development of one's own culture, and to engage
in personal or racial ancestor-seeking. The British tend to express
amusement at (for example) the American who sports a Scottish clan

tartan, or stands enraptured outside some bothy in Limerick. But even the cool British are a little impressed by titles which have been in the same family for 500 years, or by an orthodox Jew who bases his behaviour on the laws of Leviticus and Deuteronomy, and on occasions of national pomp or sentimentality they respond to the rhetoric of 'the national heritage'. If a similar rhetoric is used by Black Americans it may sometimes seem somewhat contrived but cannot be discounted. The popularity of Haley's novel *Roots* (1977) and elevation of its hero Kunta Kinte into a cult figure, testifies to a widespread interest in African history. The increasing use of the terms 'Afro-Caribbean' and 'Afro-American' is part of this movement, and the demand for 'Black Studies' and 'Black History' to be included in the British educational system should be seen in this context. Such demands come from the Caribbean rather than the Asian minority groups, since the latter have access to an unbroken historical culture in which they already take pride. Bavington has observed that there is a difference between Pathans and Punjabis in this respect. The Pathans (who were never effectively subjugated by the British Raj) are less inclined to this kind of 'paranoia' than others.

All movements that have emotional rather than rational appeal must have their extremists, but even apparent absurdities should not be dismissed unthinkingly. A West Indian who claims that 'his' people invented medicine and mathematics appears to be talking wildly until we realize that by 'his' people he means Africans, and Africa includes Egypt and, by extension, all the historical Arab cultures.

DISAPPOINTMENT IN BRITAIN

At this point we may ask, if the white man in the Caribbean was such a villain, why on earth have a quarter of a million West Indians migrated to Britain to seek their fortunes? And how could they be surprised when, on arrival, they discovered a racially stratified society here? For the West Indian islands are still riddled with colour-consciousness. In Barbados, native-born Barbadians come in every conceivable variety of colour, physiognomy, and physique. Some look as 'white' as any European, and others look purely African, but actually every Barbadian is a genetic mixture from many sources. Within one family, siblings may differ in colour by several shades, and until very recently it was a safe assumption that the lighter-skinned members would do better in life than the darker. They held administrative and commercial power, and were the most favoured marriage partners. This is changing slowly, but the social structure of Barbados — and other islands — is still stratified by colour, so how could they expect to find Britain any different?

Strangely enough, even while rebelling against 'Massa', many West Indians seem to have had at the same time a touching faith in Britain. This has been described by many writers. For example, Royer (a West Indian psychiatrist) states:

'In the aftermath of emancipation Britain became idealised in the mind of the West Indians.

The whole system of education (both formal and informal) was geared to making most West Indians believe that Great Britain was of all nations the most blessed with a love for freedom, a passion for justice.

Patriotic songs lauding the glory of Britain were taught in schools — "Rule Britannia", "Land of Hope and Glory", "The British Grenadiers".

The idea of belonging to the British Empire (upon which the sun never set) and subsequently the British Commonwealth of Nations, conjured up feelings of pride and joy which were highlighted annually on 24 May which was a great holiday set apart to foster the sense of belonging to a great community *united in bonds that transcend class and creed.*

Sports, especially cricket, and the missionary from England who was the living embodiment and constant focus of all things British, also helped to cement such attitudes.'

The West Indians who migrated to Britain were, therefore, 'confident that they were going to a land of Christians where they would be received with compassion and respect and where without much difficulty they would adjust to life and seek their fortune through employment' (Royer 1977). And this despite the bitter invective of Williams! The contradiction is not easily reconciled. Maybe in some eyes 'Massa' was one thing and Britain was another. (Williams said specifically that 'Not all Massas were white, and not all whites were Massas'.) Maybe they made the mistake of believing in the image that the British projected about themselves. Those clean-limbed and clean-living Christian sportsmen from the world of Kipling and Buchan, with their 'purity and decency', 'passion for justice', and 'love of freedom', seem quite remote from the disillusioned post-war society of Osborne and Amis into which the immigrants came: a society which finds the pomp of an imperial past, and the simple faith of its begetters, a source of embarrassment and ridicule. Whatever the reasons, the fact is that many West Indians came to Britain with high expectations of the welcome they would receive and the standards of tolerance and public morality that they would encounter. To many of that generation, secure in the certainties of their Christian faith and devout in its observances, it is not only racism but the cynicism and moral confusion of contemporary Britain that is distressing and disappointing.

WITHIN-GROUP PARANOIA

Members of minority groups may have good reason to fear hostility from the so-called 'host' population, but that is not their only problem. We have noted (Chapter 4) that an atmosphere of jealous suspicion is characteristic of peasant societies and other closed communities; and that some immigrants view the mores and customs of British society with great misgiving, making strenuous efforts to hold on to what they regard as the traditional values of their own culture (Chapter 7). In this fearful, inward-looking atmosphere, therefore, anyone who is seen to deviate too far from the accepted norm of his or her group risks being vilified or victimized by the group.

A seventeen-year-old girl who was born in Pakistan, and came to Britain at the age of seven, was seen by a psychiatrist following a suicide attempt. She was in conflict with her parents whose attitude she regarded as restrictive and repressive. She stated that she would like to leave home and make a life for herself independently. She felt unable to do so, however, *because of what would happen to her mother*. She explained that about eighteen months previously her elder sister had been in the same position and had run away from home. This action had brought disgrace on the whole family, and particularly on the girls' mother, who was severely criticized for having failed to bring up her daughter properly. She was beaten by her husband with the tacit approval of other relatives and isolated and rejected by the rest of the community. Neighbours refused to speak to her, she was insulted in the street, and refused service by one of the local shopkeepers. This 'punishment' was still going on after eighteen months. The patient felt sure that if she herself were to repeat her sister's offence her mother would be killed or commit suicide.

The story was later confirmed by her elder sister, who paid a quick and secret visit to the hospital. She had gone to live in a distant city, had changed her address three times in quick succession to evade pursuit, and dared not make any contact with her family or any member of the Pakistani community, except a tenuous·telephone contact with the patient herself. After a brief and tearful reunion in hospital, the sisters parted without recrimination, the elder to go back into hiding, and the younger to go home so that (as she put it) her mother would not be alone. Such stories are by no means unique, and by no means limited to one ethnic group. We may ask, who was being paranoid? The girl? Her sister? The father? The whole community?

REFUGEE PARANOIA

A man who had escaped from Vietnam by boat, leaving his wife and children behind, became solitary and depressed, despite the efforts of his compatriots to include him in their activities. Eventually his self-neglect was such that his worried friends brought him to see a psychiatrist. It proved quite impossible to obtain a history or elicit any information: he was initially courteous but evaded every direct question.

After the interview was over he told the interpreter that he had been very frightened by it (though he had appeared impassive). Later, it was discovered that in Vietnam he had been subjected to military inter-rogation including torture.

A woman born in Eastern Europe who came to Britain in 1945 developed in 1975 an illness for which the appropriate treatment was a course of repeated injections. Her reaction to this proposal was violent, and appeared bizarre until it was revealed that she had been in a concentration camp in which doctors were said to be carrying out experiments on prisoners by injecting noxious substances. The accusation against the camp doctors may or may not have been true but it was a common belief in the camp, so her 'paranoid' attitude to medical treatment was by no means incomprehensible. (See also Chapter 16.) It is quite possible that the high incidence of paranoia found among 'aliens' in some of the post-war studies (1–3) may have been more to do with their status as refugees than as immigrants.

NOTES

1 Own observations. A similar comment was made about West Indians in London by Kiev (1963).
2 Perhaps the most vigorous exponent of this viewpoint is Franz Fanon. See e.g. *Black Skins – White Masks* and *The Wretched of the Earth*.
3 J. T. Bavington (personal communication).

Cultural Pitfalls
in the Recognition of
Hysteria

Hysteria is a much-misused term and a dubious diagnostic category. It is employed here in the limited sense described in Appendix 1. Hysterical behaviour is motivated — albeit unconsciously — and its function is to provide a solution to a problem. For example the *malade imaginaire* who retires to a bed of sickness every time anyone in the household crosses his or her will, has found a way of controlling the household and will continue to do this as long as it is effective.

Hysterical behaviour is intended to attract attention, and influence other people — perhaps merely to elicit sympathy, or perhaps to gain some specific advantage or control. We can therefore regard hysteria as a form of communication, and in the present context that is a useful way to consider it. If the subject is fully aware of what he or she is doing (e.g. consciously feigning illness to gain an advantage) that is not hysteria but malingering. In true hysteria the subject remains unaware of the motives behind his or her behaviour and will deny any such intention vehemently. Nonetheless the motives are there, and we may be sure that the symptoms are serving a purpose in the patient's life. The boundary between hysteria and malingering (conscious or unconscious motivation) is not hard and fast.

Hysteria is the most culturally variable of all conditions. To be an effective means of communication, the message must be transmitted in a 'language' that will attract attention and obtain the required response. In Freud's own practice pseudo-epileptic fits, or dramatic paralysis of a limb, or loss of the power of speech, were apparently quite common. In contemporary British practice these are rare: the preferred attention-seeking behaviour is a sequence of chronic or recurrent ailments (for which of course, no organic cause can ever be found).

Hysteria can mimic any physical disorder, known or unknown, and the greater the medical knowledge the better the mimicry. (Hysterical

nurses can be very convincing, and hysterical doctors pose terrible diagnostic problems.) Possibly Freud's patients mimicked epilepsy or paralysis because in those days untreated epileptics and cripples were more
commonly encountered, a part of everyone's life experience. Hysteria
can also mimic other kinds of mental disease. Thus we may have
hysterical pseudo-dementia, *hysterical phobias*, or *hysterical pseudo-
psychoses*.

HYSTERICAL PSEUDO-PSYCHOSIS ('HYSTERICAL MADNESS')

A fifteen-year-old Pakistani girl was referred to a child psychiatrist
because of disruptive behaviour in the classroom, and visual hallucinations. She described the appearance of strange small figures, variously
described as 'spirits' and 'fairies', which she perceived dancing about
the room in front of her. The description of these apparitions was clear
and detailed, she said that they beckoned to her and she was obliged
to act on their instructions. From time to time she had 'collapsed' in
a dramatic fashion, and had something like an epileptic fit. Her eyes
rolled, she uttered nonsense, and behaved in a violent, uncontrolled
manner for a few minutes, after which she slowly returned to normal
and claimed no recollection of the event. Her parents were convinced
that she was afflicted with some kind of 'madness', for which they were
inclined to find a supernatural explanation.

Such behaviour would be rare in an English adolescent girl, but it is
not all that uncommon in Pakistan[1] and many other cultures. It usually
turns out that the girl has some problem or conflict on her mind that
she cannot express openly, or which she feels other people are not taking
sufficiently seriously. In this case it was a matter of pressure to achieve
academic results which were beyond her, combined with a somewhat
repressive attitude by her parents.

What would an English girl have done in that situation? One possibility
is that she would have taken an overdose and been admitted to hospital
as a case of attempted suicide. This kind of suicidal gesture – sometimes
called 'parasuicide' because there is no real intention to kill oneself –
is an extremely popular attention-seeking manoeuvre in contemporary
British society, sometimes described as a modern epidemic. The patients
always say that they are 'depressed', but only a small minority are
suffering from a depressive illness in the sense defined in Appendix 1:
usually it is a 'cry for help'. Both these girls are doing the same thing.
Each is making a dramatic gesture that signals the message 'I can't
cope', and in either case they might be doing it consciously or unconsciously or half-and-half. They have both chosen to make their
point by behaving in a way that will ensure attention.

Considering hysteria as a form of communication, we can perhaps understand the reasons for the difference. It is partly a matter of the girl's own concept of 'mental illness', which is based on what they have heard and seen in other people, and it is partly a matter of impact. We have already noted that in Pakistani village culture, as in many others, 'madness' in the family is a major disaster. It is highly stigmatized, and has consequences for other family members. A teenage girl who exhibits signs of madness is certain to get the rest of the family rushing about in alarm and paying a lot of attention to her needs, which they might not have done if she had merely sat in a corner looking gloomy. The opposite applies to the English girl: if she spoke of seeing fairies she might just be told not to be silly, whereas we have our own cultural taboos and hangups about death, and particularly suicide.[2]

The practical significance of this is that because hallucinations, convulsions, or wildly excited behaviour are not often included in the repertoire of hysteria in Britain, they take the British practitioner unawares and are likely to be misdiagnosed as psychotic. It is not unknown for a British patient to produce symptoms of schizophrenia purely as an hysterical mechanism, so the diagnostic problem does occasionally arise; but it is an unusual choice of symptoms, and the person whose hysteria takes that form instead of some more common-place pattern is often a rather odd personality (unless he or she is copying it from someone close to them – as in *'folie a deux'*) and may well develop a truly schizophrenic illness at a later stage. This is not true of hysterical pseudo-psychosis in Asian, African or Afro-Caribbean patients where the resemblance to psychosis is purely a diagnostic red herring, and the correct diagnosis, treatment, and prognosis, treatment, and prognosis is that of hysteria.[3] The teenage girl's hallucinations (in our Pakistani example above) should be treated in the same way as her English counterpart's overdose.

We can now add some more sections to our nosological diagram. (*Table 14(1)*. This way of visualizing it may serve as a diagnostic aide-memoire for some syndromes which, though rarely seen in Britain, can certainly exist in other cultures.

HYSTERIA AND ROLE-PLAYING

The diagnosis of hysteria is made partly on the pattern of symptoms and on the discovery of their motivation, but also partly on the *manner* in which those symptoms are presented. A patient who enters the surgery clutching his abdomen and beseeching the doctor to do something instantly about the agonizing pain which cannot be tolerated for another moment, but is seen immediately before or after the consultation

Table 14 (1)

	Depression	*Excitement*	*Schiz . . .*
ENDOGENOUS Biological, genetic factors. Stress not primary cause. ↑ | | | ↓	**1** *'Endogenous depression'* (psychotic depression). Recognized in all cultures, but symptoms may differ.	**3** *'Mania'* Recognized in all cultures. Less common than depression.	**5** *'Schizophrenia'* Probably exists everywhere.
REACTIVE Response to stress, conflict, 'Neurotic' rather than 'psychotic'. ↑ | | | ↓	**2** *'Reactive depression'* Common in Britain. In other cultures may be regarded as not being a 'medical' problem.	**4** *'Reactive excitation'* ('reactive mania'). Rare among British but well known elsewhere. Psychogenic psychoses.	**6** *'Actue Schiz-ophreniform stress reaction'*
HYSTERICAL Motivated, attention-seeking.	**7** (e.g. many cases of 'parasuicide') Common in Britain. Rare in some other cultures.	**8** Varieties of *'Hysterical Madness'* (hysterical pseudo-psychosis). Uncommon among British. More common in non-European cultures.	**9**

chatting happily to a neighbour or waiting calmly at the bus stop, may be said to be 'putting it on a bit' for the doctor's benefit. This is likely to be taken as evidence of hysteria or at least a somewhat hysterical personality. But this analysis contains another cultural pitfall.

An Indian woman who visits a friend to offer condolences on a recent bereavement might be observed walking cheerfully up to the door: but when ushered into the presence of the bereaved she might burst into loud lamentations in which she would be joined by the widow and other women of the family. Five minutes later they may be sitting together quite composedly sipping tea. The outburst of emotion was not hysterical, nor was it necessarily insincere: but it had about it something of the nature of a *ritual*: it was the proper and socially expected behaviour, the appropriate role for the situation. To behave in any other way would be a social solecism.

So it is when visiting the doctor: one does not waste the doctor's time with trivialities. The consultation is a serious and formal situation for which there are appropriate formuli of behaviour. But whereas to the British, formality usually tends towards clipped understatement, in many cultures formality may equally include elements of over-statement — and this should not be construed as hysterical, nor as an indicator of sincerity or the severity of the complaint.

HYPOCHONDRIASIS, HYSTERIA, AND SOMATIZATION

A familiar figure in the doctor's surgery is the sad-looking middle-aged Asian man who turns up with one minor ailment or complaint after another. He often looks about seventy years old but his 'passport age'[4] is quite a lot less. There is little or nothing wrong with him physically, but he seems determined to be an invalid. He is regarded as an hysterical hypochondriac, and everyone gets fed up with him.

It is possible that he is suffering from a depressive illness, and somatizing his distress in the way described in Chapter 10; this diagnostic pitfall should always be kept firmly in mind. It may be, however, that he has a social role problem. He has reached a time of life at which had he remained in his traditional culture he could relax into the secure status of a patriarch — respected, obeyed, and waited on by his family. In Britain he is expected to go on working (probably at a heavy labouring job), and his domestic authority is constantly challenged (see Chapter 7). In this predicament, the role of an invalid may be the only legitimate role available to him. If only he would admit this to his doctor, and say that he felt depressed, his complaints would make diagnostic sense: but as a hypochondriac, a surgery-haunter, exaggerator-of-trivia, and persistent sick-note-requester, he gets off on the wrong foot. He compounds his offence by over-dramatizing, instead of displaying the stoicism that might gain him some grudging sympathy.

The stereotype of *Asian Hypochondriasis* is reinforced by two other factors. There are a few immigrants — a small minority — who are so delighted with the benevolence of the welfare state that they see it as a cornucopia which it would be a shame not to utilize to the full. Every traveller in Asia soon becomes accustomed to the hordes of beggars who importune passers-by with heart-rendering tales of distress, and of course this kind of begging does not carry the same kind of stigma everywhere that it does in Northern Europe. The vast majority of immigrants to Britain are not importunate, and do not set out to get as much as they can out of the State, but inevitably there are a few exceptions, and they create a lot of ill-feeling.

The other point is that many Asians in Britain do not know that they can obtain medicine for minor ailments over the counter from a local chemist, without a prescription. They tend therefore to consult general practitioners for colds, digestive upsets and other minor ailments that most English families would treat themselves with proprietory medicines (Aslam *et al.* in press; Walker, Aslam, and Davis 1980).

NOTES

1 I am indebted to Dr Ahmed Ali of Peshawar for the aphorism: 'Hallucinations in Britain – think about schizophrenia: hallucinations in Pakistan – think first about hysteria'.

2 Adolescents who wish to assert their independence *vis-a-vis* their parents commonly 'challenge' them on one or two specific issues. In any particular family, the arena of battle may be clothes, coming home late, or hairstyles, and we may say that this particular battleground has been chosen by mutual agreement, since it would not be a battleground unless both sides chose to make it one. Most parents are ruefully aware that their children are skilful at selecting battlegrounds on which they (the parents) have a weak position because of their own uncertainties, fears, or inconsistencies. Parents who have over-valued, confused or neurotic attitudes to money or sex or social prestige are likely to be challenged by their adolescent children on money, sex, or social prestige respectively. The choice is not usually a conscious one: it 'just happens'. Using this as a model, we may speculate on the choice of symptoms which distressed people select to challenge the societies in which they live. In Freud's Vienna, sexual hypocrisy was built in to the culture and therefore sexuality was an obvious subject for hysteria. In contemporary Britain the great taboo subjects are death (which as a culture we handle very badly) and aggression (of which we are afraid) so we have epidemics of overdoses and vandalism. In cultures where there is a superstitious dread of 'insanity' we may expect to find hysterical madness.

3 Very similar observations have been made among Puerto Rican adolescents in New York:

> 'the incidence of schizophrenia among Puerto Ricans appears high partly because of lack of understanding of cultural phenomena. I submit . . . that many hysterical dissociative episodes, especially among adolescent Puerto Ricans, have been misdiagnosed as schizophenia.'   (Rendon 1976 : 170)

4 Because birth certificates are not issued routinely in many parts of rural India and Pakistan, an Indian or Pakistani may not be able to state his age exactly, and when applying for travel documents to enter Britain he may have made an approximate guess. In some cases, he may have deliberately underestimated his age to improve his prospects of entry. The age recorded on his passport is his official age as far as the British authorities are concerned and there is no way it can be changed retrospectively. Hence a man may be over seventy, but if his passport says he is not yet sixty-five he cannot draw a pension.

15

Culture-Bound Syndromes

Researchers in various prescientific societies have recorded examples of mental disorders which are not easily fitted in to the European classification system and have been thought to be specific to a particular culture. They have been called *culture-bound syndromes*, and they include *Amuk, Banga, Jiryan, Koro, Latah, Negi-negi, Misala, Piblokto, Susto*, and *Windigo*.[1] These names contribute a touch of exotic spice to the British psychiatric text-book, but their importance to the practitioner is minimal. According to Kiev: 'Culture-bound disorders are for the most part variants of the severe functional psychoses and of various neurotic syndromes . . . These are not new diagnostic entities: they are in fact similar to those already known in the West' (Kiev 1972). In fact, some of them appear to be merely the local name for mental disorder of any kind (e.g. *Banga, Misala*). Others refer to ascribed cause: e.g. *Susto* (Latin American) means temporary loss of the soul from the body as a result of stress, and is therefore an explanation for illness rather than a syndrome. *Windigo psychosis* (North America) appears to be a form of severe depression in which culturally-determined fears of cannibalism colour the depressive delusions. Supernatural and animistic attributes of mental illness are common and they take local forms in different cultures. (See Chapter 13.) Where the difference is one of behaviour rather than explanation, it may often be a local variant of psychogenic psychosis or hysteria (see Chapters 11, 12 and 14).

There is no universal agreement about *Amuk, Latah, Piblokto*. *Amuk* is an outburst of murderous frenzy that occurs in South East Asia and has been variously attributed to drug intoxication, psychogenic psychosis, and schizophrenia. *Latah* (Malaysia) is probably a culture-bound form of hysteria. *Piblokto* (Eskimo women) has features of agitated depression and fugue-like withdrawal (Kiev 1972).

Koro and *Jiryan* are psychosexual disorders. *Koro* patients have the delusional fear that the penis will retract into the abdomen and thereby cause death. It would not be surprising to discover cases of Koro among the Chinese community in Britain but we are not aware of any published report. Yap has offered a psychodynamic interpretation of it in terms of Chinese concepts of sexuality and the balance of Yin and Yang (Yap 1964). *Jiryan* is a common complaint in Pakistan and also in India where it is alternatively called the *Dhat* syndrome. It consists of a fixed belief that sperm is leaking from the body in the urine (Carstairs 1956). In some cases the patient may be misled by the cloudiness of his urine due to urates, prostatic secretion, or chronic infection, but it is not essential to have any objective evidence to support the belief and it is usually held with firm conviction, inaccessible to reasoned argument. There is a cultural belief that 'it takes forty drops of blood to make one drop of semen', and since both blood and semen are non-renewable sources obviously any wastage is a matter for concern.[2] The complaint of *Jiryan/Dhat* is often made by young men who have anxieties about their potency or guilt-feelings about masturbation. It may also be used as an explanation for disorders in which the cause is not primarily sexual, e.g. a man with weakness, general malaise and debility due to depression or to an organic disease, may attribute his symptoms to *Jiryan* in the same way that an English patient might attribute them to constipation.

NOTES

1 For more details of culture-bound syndromes refer to Kiev (1972) Yap (1951) or Lipsedge and Littlewood (1979). The last includes a careful review of current thinking and an exhaustive bibliography.
2 See 'Concept of Limited Good', Chapter 4.

Refugees

The psychological reactions of refugees require a separate note, because while they share many of the problems of other migrants, they differ in two important respects: their experiences before reaching safety — which are to do with violence, trauma, and loss — and their reception and resettlement on arrival.

We must not generalize too readily about 'refugees' as a category, since there are great differences in the culture from which they came, and their reasons for leaving. The Displaced Persons who settled in Britain in the immediate post-war years (Poles, Ukrainians, Byelorussians, Latvians, Lithuanians, Estonians, and a few from other European and Balkan countries) had been separated from their homelands by war and had spent years in labour camps or concentration camps before being liberated (see Chapter 3, p. 26). They were mostly young adults, more men than women, unmarried or forcibly parted from their wives; they spanned every socio-economic class, some being aristocrats or intellectuals, others with the characteristics of peasants (as described in Chapter 4). The Hungarians who followed them in 1956 were also, predominantly, young men. They were not a cross-section of Hungarian society, but included a good many who had been in conflict with the authorities in their country for either political or criminal activities and seized the opportunity to emigrate during the brief period that the frontier was open. Not surprisingly, they exhibited different kinds of psychiatric problems from their predecessors; a significant number had pre-existing psychiatric illness or personality problems (Eitinger 1960; Eitinger and Grünfield 1966; Mezey 1960a). The Czechs who escaped after the abortive 'Prague Spring' of 1967 included a large number with academic and professional backgrounds.

For the Cypriots and Ugandan Asians the situation was different because there was a community of compatriots already established in Britain, forming an enclave into which the newcomers could be welcomed. The Cypriots were rapidly absorbed into the existing Cypriot community; and the Ugandan Asians despite a determined effort by the Government to disperse them throughout Britain managed in a few years to 'home in' on those cities (e.g. Leicester) that already had Gujerati communities. Unlike the examples mentioned earlier, the Cypriots and Ugandan Asians came as families — in the latter case the whole community was expelled, including young and old, fit and unfit, mentally stable and unstable together. The refugees from Chile, Argentina, and other Latin American countries included a large number of political activists who fled to escape the firing squad often having experienced imprisonment and torture because of their political beliefs; many of them had been leaders in their own society, and regarded their period of exile as a part of the ongoing political struggle, to which they would return. The 13,000 Vietnamese who have arrived in the last two years have suffered perhaps the greatest cultural displacement of all with no political or cultural unanimity to sustain group cohesion and no pre-existing ethnic community to cushion their adaptation.

In addition to these groups who have arrived at particular times, there are individuals from many other countries who have sought asylum in Britain after escaping secretly from political or economic oppression, or in some cases having come as students and found that changes in their own country made it unsafe for them to return. These *individuals* may experience a greater sense of isolation than those who arrive in groups. Do these differences invalidate any conclusions about 'the refugee experience', or can we make any generalizations? It would be helpful to do so if possible, because there will certainly be other refugee crises in future and up to now each has been dealt with on an *ad hoc* basis. Each time an emergency arises teams of workers come into existence, locally and nationally: apart from the permanent staff of the refugee organizations (who are so few in number that they can only have an advisory or administrative role), most workers have had no previous experience of similar situations. The team may contain practitioners in various disciplines and volunteers who come forward motivated by religious or humanitarian concern, or political sympathy. Some of these volunteers may be former compatriots of the refugees able to instruct on cultural aspects. Few if any will know about refugees *as such*. Each team learns as it goes along and is in danger of repeating the mistakes of its predecessors.

PREDICTABLE PROBLEMS

The administrative requirements of Resettlement Centres, and the problems of diet, documentation, interpreting and medical services, are outside the scope of this book. What about mental and emotional problems?

We may safely assume that out of any large group of refugees, some will develop severe emotional problems or overt mental illness. To ask how many is not a useful question, since this will depend on the availability of psychiatric services and their acceptability, and other kinds of support available. Availability will be affected by the presence of mental health specialists who can speak the right language. Acceptability is influenced by three factors at least:

(1) Attitudes to mental illness in the culture of origin and its stigma (discussed in more detail in Chapter 18).
(2) People who have suffered torture and 'brain washing' may view any professionals with suspicion.
(3) The staff who are responsible for the day-to-day care of refugees may be reluctant to call in psychiatric help because they are predisposed to regard the refugees as tough, resilient, admirable people who have survived unimaginable hazards and can cope, or because they perceive it as their own job to cope and regard any breakdowns as their failure.

In terms of epidemiology, therefore, referral statistics are unreliable, and there is no point in trying to distinguish between *severe adaptation problems* on the one hand and *mental disorder* on the other.

Can we identify *who* are likely to be 'at risk'? Kunz (1973) divides patterns of flight into *anticipatory* and *acute* — and believes that the latter group (who lack time to prepare) will have the greater problems. American organizations working with Indo-Chinese refugees report that the age group nineteen to thirty-five is most at risk, but depression and anxiety are also common in the thirty-six to fifty-five age group where there is a loss of role and status (Pennsylvania Department of Public Welfare Report 1979). Rahe and colleagues (1978) identified women aged between twenty and forty as the most disturbed in an American settlement camp for Vietnamese. After reviewing the literature, Stein (1980) picks out single people, and those separated from their families. Nguyen (1980) comments on the vulnerability of those who travel alone, but also mentions (in the context of South-East Asian culture) nuclear family units that are separated from their extended family networks. We might predict that those who had experienced the most severe deprivation and the deaths of close relatives, would be the more depressed, but it may be that it is even harder to have left one's family behind and be uncertain what has befallen them. 'Survivor Guilt' (see below) may afflict those who have *not* had a very bad time personally.

When do most problems arise? Organizations surveyed by the

Pennsylvania questionnaire concluded that problems tend to surface 'some years' after arrival, and this view is taken by Krumperman (1981) Bram (personal communication), Montero (1980), and others, and accords with the present author's own experience of Uganda Asians, Chileans, and Vietnamese. Tyhurst (1977) is prepared to be very precise about this:

'The first and most significant component of the clinical picture which is relevant for the planning of assistance to refugees is the *predictable onset* of general personal disequilibrium . . . which reaches its peak at about six months after entry.'

(Tyhurst 1977 : 323, her italics)

The experience of Tyhurst and her colleagues spans thirty years and includes the resettlement in Canada of post-war European refugees, Hungarians, Czechs, and Uganda Asians in turn, so the observations made by this team deserve respect. She continues:

'This period of turmoil is preceded by an . . . "incubation" period, over the first one to two months after entry. At this time, the person feels energetic, in good spirits, even euphoric; the only problem which regularly presents itself is catastrophic dreaming revolving around the experiences of danger and flight . . . alerting those who care for refugees of the predictable difficulties that lie ahead will "normalize" the perception of these phenomena."

(Tyhurst 1977 : 323)

Other workers have noticed this 'honeymoon period' but not everyone agrees about the predictable nature and timing of the reactive 'disequilibrium' that follows: there are too many variables. Those who spend months in transit camps or settlement camps are in a different position from those who do not; and in the case of, for example, a Vietnamese who spent months in camp in Hong Kong, then further months in one in Scotland, and has now been given a house in a British city, *but really wanted to go to Canada, where his relatives are*, there is an obvious difference between 'reaching safety' and 'reaching one's destination'. A political exile who plans to return may not regard Britain as a 'destination' at all (Munoz 1980). It may be only after leaving the settlement camp and entering the host society, and learning its language that the refugee learns about society's ambivalence to him, and realizes that everyone is not so well-disposed as the refugee workers he has been with so far.

What kinds of emotional reactions can we predict? Tyhurst has delineated a 'Social Displacement Syndrome' of which the symptoms are:

(1) *Paranoid behaviour* ranging from attitudes of suspicion and vigilance to acute paranoid psychotic episodes.

(2) *Generalized hypochondriasis* with the tendency to shift complaints from system to system.

(3) *Anxiety and depression* usually somatized, coupled with 'inability to describe' the emotion as such.

(4) *Disorientation and confusion* varying from day to day, and including misidentification, e.g.:

> 'Many D.P. patients insisted that they had seen their parents among the medical personnel, or the Nazi labour camp commanders among the officials of the Department of Labour . . . at times there were acute confusional states with vivid hallucinations and illusions . . . these receded after a few days of hospitalisation . . . '   (Tyhurst 1977 : 325)

(5) *'Desocialization'*: Tyhurst states that some loss of social competence is characteristic of all refugees, but those who have been living under unnatural social conditions for long periods are likely to have definite impairment in their abilities to relate, and this is shown in their attitudes to each other and to helpers and officials.

Stein (1980) has a rather similar list, and adds: *Emotional outbursts of anger and crying.* Rahe (1978) reported 'gross behavioural disturbance' as a feature of the first few months, replaced later by anxiety, depression, and apathy. Alcoholism has been mentioned as a problem in several reports.

The *aggressiveness* of refugees has been noted by several writers and may pose a particular problem for volunteer workers untrained in social casework. Stein points out that the aggressiveness that produces negative effects in violence, crime, and suicide, may also be the basis of innovative, risk-taking 'independent' behaviour, and makes the further interesting point that the *survival strategies* that have enabled the refugee to 'beat the system' during his incarceration or flight, may become habitual and cause behaviour which, in the new situation, is criticized as antisocial and ungrateful. Stein also refers to feelings of *invulnerability*.

Krumperman (1981) and Davidson (1979a, 1979b) have both emphasized that one of the ways for an individual to defend himself against the psychological consequences of overwhelming disaster is to shut off all emotional responses and become 'psychically numbed' or 'armour plated'. Such a person is unable to enter into warm empathic relationships with new people, and may not be able to maintain the relationships which he already has — e.g. with wife or children. Several writers have listed marital conflicts as common problems. In such a case the practitioner or refugee worker may feel intuitively that the victim is 'choked' by his emotions, and be sympathetic: but may later come to believe that this person *has no emotions* (which is, in a sense the case, since all emotions have been banished from consciousness); and if other undesirable, antisocial, paranoid, or aggressive behaviour is displayed (as above) the victim may be stigmatized as an unpleasant, cold, callous, or selfish person, who does not merit sympathy after all.

PREVENTION AND MANAGEMENT

The question of how to cope with these emotional problems belongs properly in Part IV, but can more conveniently be considered here. The allocation of resources will be determined by the scale of the problem and extent of public sympathy. The Hungarians arrived at a time when many of the British public were aghast at the Russian invasion of Hungary, and morally dismayed by Britain's recent intervention in Suez, which they saw as contributory to it. The refugee organizations were deluged by offers of assistance, and there were few problems of placement (Pearce, personal communication). The Ugandan Asians, on the other hand, attracted some of the prevailing hostility against Asian immigrants in general. The Vietnamese attracted a lot of goodwill because of extensive media coverage of their sufferings, but that did not prevent the National Front from demonstrating against them, and even in America, where some collective responsibility was felt for events in Vietnam,

> 'many Americans feared that an influx of refugees would create an added drain on already over-burdened public assistance rolls. . . a 1975 Gallup Poll . . . reported that 54 per cent of Americans felt the Vietnamese should not be permitted to stay in this country.'
> (Montero 1979 : 625)

It is likely that the team attempting resettlement will have to work under pressure and with inadequate resources, and will be unable to mobilize enough skilled personnel to cope as well as they would wish with the emotional problems that arise. It is essential to involve local resources including the primary health care teams and Social Service Departments as well as volunteers (Tyhurst 1977; Phillips and Pearson 1981). Because of practical and emotional pressures in the situation, practitioners from different disciplines may experience more than usual difficulty in working together.

From the reports quoted above and others, there seems to be general agreement on three principles of refugee resettlement. The first is that organized camps, hostels, and similar transitional institutions, which are undoubtedly useful places for sorting out immediate administrative problems and providing language classes, ought to be used for as short a period as possible. The better organized the camp, the more it resembles a 'total institution' and induces dependency, apathy, and learned helplessness. This can be mitigated by democratization, insisting that the residents share as fully as possible in decision making, and creating as far as possible the atmosphere of a therapeutic community. In such an atmosphere it may be possible for refugees to share their experiences and feelings with each other and with the staff.

The second principle is that dispersal policies increase the problems of individuals, and it at all possible they should be rehoused in places where an ethnic or cultural community already exists, or in such concentration that one can come into being. The adaptational problems are not all overcome in the first six or twelve months; they may be still to come, and the evidence is clear that isolated individuals and families are at greatest risk of breakdown. A permanent organization, social centre, or team of workers with which refugees can maintain contact for as long as necessary, would be a highly desirable resource, and might provide the base of a continuing sense of group cohesion (COLAT 1981).

These two principles are to some extent contradictory. There are no ideal solutions, and practical constraints usually determine policies. The third principle, which may help to bridge the contradiction, is to make full use of key people within the group itself. Tyhurst points out that 'The capacity of man to give is often denied the refugee, who is assigned a place at the receiving end of society' (Tyhurst 1977 : 341). Nguyen (1980) calls for training of mental health workers within the community and the creation of comprehensive community support systems, and recommends the active participation of skilled people inside the group in every aspect of the resettlement process, and the employment of 'bicultural' staff. Stein (1980) states that

> 'In most refugee programmes there is a reluctance to perceive a shift in the refugee's role and accept them as participants in their own resettlement . . . Most agencies and co-ordinating councils exclude the bilingual staff from policy decision making.'
>
> (Stein 1980 : 112)

In the longer term, he believes that the refugee community itself should become an important aid resource. The practice of training suitably qualified people within the group, and employing them as settlement workers, has not been tried extensively in Britain, but it was adopted in 1981 on a small scale by the Save the Children Fund, Refugee Action, and British Refugee Council.

LONG-TERM PROBLEMS

Because there has been no differentiation between refugees and other groups of immigrants in Britain, we do not know about the statistics of mental illness in later years, but the findings of Murphy (1955) agree with those in other countries and suggest a continuing vulnerability (Eitinger and Grünfeld 1966, Eitinger and Schwarz 1981, Krupinski *et al.* 1973). Schizophrenia appears to be the commonest diagnosis in all reports (but the reliability of this diagnosis is questioned elsewhere in this book). Krupinski makes an interesting observation that Jews, despite having experienced the most severe persecution of any of the groups he studied in Australia, have lower subsequent breakdown rates than other refugees, although still twice that of the indigenous population for males, and four times that for females. The others had even higher rates:

> 'The second most severely persecuted group, the Poles, Russians and Ukrainians, showed high rates of psychiatric disorders and these were proportionate to the severity of their war experiences. They came from low, mostly peasant, social backgrounds and they have remained in unskilled and semi-skilled occupations in Australia.
>   The third group . . . from Baltic countries, Czechoslovakia, Hungary and Yugoslavia . . . suffered least from Nazi persecutions and, in most cases, they had left their countries before the communist takeover. They came predominantly from a middle-class background and showed a significant downward mobility in Australia. Their high rates of psychiatric disturbances were not related to their war experiences but were associated rather with the loss of social status and the stresses of migration.
>   There were significant symptom-free periods in most cases . . . their illnesses could be regarded as late sequelae of persecution or migration stresses. Neither family support, not the degree of assimilation in Australia, seemed to have any protective influence on the refugees.   (Krupinski *et al.* 1973 : 47)

Bram (1979) contrasts the lives of Polish doctors, who were licensed to practice in Britain, with lawyers and army officers, who were forced into unskilled employment.

We cannot, however, discount the effects of the traumatic experience itself. Krumperman and his colleagues in Holland find evidence that violence, disaster, and bereavement can all produce long-term consequences (Krumperman 1981), and they draw specific attention to the effects of torture and rape. Davidson has followed up a large number of

concentration camp survivors in Israel, and finds that their apparently
satisfactory adaptation can break down after many years (Davidson
1979a, 1979b, 1980a, 1980b). Survivor guilt is a common feature, revolving around the unanswerable question 'Why was *I* permitted to live
when so many others did not?' Krumperman, Davidson, Munoz and
others discuss exile as a form of bereavement, and this concept opens up
useful insights and lines of therapy. After bereavement, mourning is an essential and therapeutic process, and the task of the therapist is to help
the victim to mourn (Freud 1917). But faced by total disaster, with loss
of *all* loved ones, and of country, complete dissociation from the past,
destruction of all the external resources that a bereaved person might
use to reconstruct an identity, loss of commonality (in Davidson's
phrase); then the task may be too great to be faced, and mourning — or
sufficient mourning — may not take place immediately or at all. The
'inappropriate' outburst of grief or anger, unexplained episodes of
depression, and emotional over-reactions to comparatively minor
disappointments at a later stage, can be understood as ways of releasing
some of the repressed internal emotion in 'manageable' quantities. The
interpretation offered by Davidson and supported by Bram (personal
communications), is that *people will find opportunities* for further
mourning as and when they can. These two clinicians have had immense
experience in the long-term follow-up of survivors, and this seems a
particularly helpful and positive insight.

PROBLEMS OF THE ELDERLY

Bram (1979), Hitch and Rack (1980), and Jagucki (1981) have all
drawn attention to the position of elderly exiles who have to re-enact
the refugee experience at the end of their lives. (See Chapter 7, p. 86.)

CHILDREN

Most authorities state that children survive the refugee experience better
than adults, as long as their parents are with them. Vasquez (1981)
however points out that:

> 'for some young people the trauma of exile is crystallised in their
> school situation. School is seen as an extension of the repression
> that exists in their own countries, causing a mental block against
> studies or a wholesale rejection of school.'   (Vasquez 1981 : 27)

Vasquez gives quite a gloomy picture of the adjustment problems in
the (Latin American) adolescents she studied. Research by the Comité
Inter-Mouvement Auprès des Evacués, Paris, suggests that relation-

ships between children and their parents may be damaged more than is apparent on the surface (CIMADE 1981). Krupinski states that

> 'a quarter of the children of the patient group of refugees were reported to have significant psychiatric problems. These are likely to constitute a psychiatrically vulnerable group in the Australian population.'   (Krupinski *et al*. 1973 : 47)

This supports the unconfirmed impression that the children of post-war refugees in Britain have experienced more than average behavioural problems in adolescence and early adulthood.

NOTE

1 For background data on refugees see Murphy (1955); Beijer, in Jackson (1969); Zwingmann and Pfister-Ammende (1973); D'Souza (1980).

Epidemiology

Bearing in mind all the diagnostic pitfalls we may doubt the validity of statistics about the prevalence of mental disorders in different cultural groups. Berger expresses this with characteristic vigour:

'It is absurd to consider the health of migrant workers as though they were healthy or sick like others. Their function, the conditions of their presence here, are incompatible with the norms of preventive and clinical medicine. The norms do not apply to them. In France surveys have shown that the ratio of mental illness among immigrants is two or three times higher than among French citizens. But the category of mental illness is suspect. It would be more, not less scientific to say that immigrants suffer twice or three times as much from insecurity and unhappiness.'   (Berger and Mohr 1975 : 147)

Nonetheless, the question is frequently asked whether immigrants have rates of psychiatric illness that differ from the rest of the population. If it were possible to make accurate estimates the information would be valuable for at least two reasons:

'For the social scientist, immigration provides an unparallelled opportunity to study the effects of social change on mental health. The clinician, on the other hand, is concerned about the immigrant's need for special services: to the degree that immigrants constitute a high-risk group for mental illness, they may require more of different health and social services.'   (Roskies 1978 : 4)

Epidemiological studies have proliferated in many parts of the world. Some of them seem to show that immigrants are a high risk group, including the pioneer studies in America (Malzberg 1935; Ødegaard 1932, 1936), Scandinavia (Eitinger 1959; Astrup and Ødegaard 1960), and Australia (Krupinski *et al.* 1965, 1973, 1975). Other surveys, however, have revealed an unexpectedly low prevalence rate (Murphy 1965a).

(Reviews of the literature have been provided by Sanua (1969), Murphy (1973b) Lipsedge and Littlewood (1979), and Eitinger (1981), among others.) However, each migrant group is different, not only in its culture of origin and the reception it receives, but in demography, age-structure, and motives for migrating. The distinction between settlers, refugees, and *Gastarbeiters* (see Chapter 3) is crucial, but not always sufficiently recognized. It is dangerous, therefore, to extrapolate from one set of figures to another.

The research carried out in Britain post-war has been reviewed comprehensively elsewhere (Bagley 1968, 1975; Brandon 1979; Rack 1982). Most of the epidemiological reports depend on either hospital admission figures or general practice data. Several small studies published in the 1960s seemed to show high morbidity rates among West-Indian born subjects (Pinsent 1963; Kiev 1963, 1964, 1965; Gordon 1965; Hemsi 1967), and Asian subjects (Hashmi 1966, 1968; Bagley 1969, 1971a, 1972; Giggs 1973; Pinto 1974b). High rates for Eastern European refugees were reported after the war (Murphy 1955) and again recently (Hitch and Rack 1980). Most of the early studies are open to criticism on the grounds of small sample size, and insufficient attention to variables of age, sex, and social class. (New Commonwealth immigrants included a disproportionate number of young adults, males in particular among Asians, so the comparative figures have to be age-related and sex-related to be meaningful.)

HOSPITAL ADMISSION RATES

Some larger-scale surveys of hospital-admission data have become available in the last few years. Cochrane (1977) has analysed the figures for England and Wales in 1971, and Hitch (1975) Carpenter and Brockington (1980) and Dean and his colleagues (1981) have calculated the first-admissions data for Bradford, Manchester, and South-East England respectively. Cochrane obtained admission figures for all mental hospitals in England and Wales for 1971 and compared these with the 1971 census data on place of birth. Birthplace was recorded in only 70 per cent of patients and the assumption was made that most of the remainder were in fact British-born. Having corrected for age/sex variables, Cochrane found that the admission rates were higher than indigenous for Irish, Polish, and Scots immigrants, low for Indians and Pakistanis, and approximately the same for the Caribbean-born. (Cochrane 1977).

The other three surveys were limited to *first-time admissions* only, and are not therefore comparable with Cochrane's findings (since in most British psychiatric hospitals readmissions account for 30–60 per cent of all admissions). Each has used a different technique of age/sex standardization, and ethnic classification, and there are quite marked differences in the total (or British-born) rates which they report, presumably reflecting local differences in resources and admissions policy. In order to obtain some rough comparability, the figures which are provided in each report have been converted to a percentage of the British-born base-rate figures given in the same report, and this comparison is summarized in *Table 17 (1)* (for New Commonwealth immigrants only). It will be seen that the rates for West Indians are about one-and-a-half times the indigenous rate and the rates for women are a little higher than those of men. In the case of Asian patients, there are some seemingly irreconcilable contradictions. Cochrane found low rates in both Indians and Pakistanis. Hitch found a significantly high rate in Pakistani women but not in Indians. Dean and his colleagues report the exact reverse, with significantly high rates for Indians but low rates for Pakistanis, while Carpenter and Brockington did not discriminate between the two nationalities but recorded significantly high rates for the Asian group as a whole (see *Table 17 (1)*).

None of these differences comes near the 500 per cent differences found by some post-war workers among refugees, (Eitinger 1959; Eitinger and Grünfeld 1966) and it would be wise to keep in mind Murphy's advice:

> 'The correct contribution of epidemiology in this field should not be the production of spuriously precise rates, but the elucidation of probable patterns and relationships between sociocultural variables, when these relationships are difficult to perceive clinically.'
>
> (Murphy 1965b)

At present it is probably fair to say that no consistent trends can be detected, and such differences as exist cannot be explained by any simple generalization.

FACTORS THAT MAY CAUSE ILLNESS

Pinto (1974a) collected socio-economic data on forty-eight Asian patients in London and a comparison group of Asian non-patients, and reported that the patients were more isolated, had worse housing conditions, and had suffered greater loss of economic status than the non-patients. Bagley (1971b) compared twenty-seven West Indians diagnosed as schizophrenic with twenty-seven English schizophrenics and twenty-seven West Indians with no psychiatric disorders. He found that both groups of West Indians had more 'chronic environmental stress' than the English. The West Indian patients differed from West Indian

Summary of admissions data

Table 17 (1)

Country of birth	England and Wales 1971 (Cochrane 1977) All admissions		Bradford 1968-70 (Hitch 1975)		Manchester 1973-75 (Carpenter and Brockington 1980) First admissions only		South-East England 1976 (Dean et al. 1981)	
	Male	Female	Male	Female	Male	Female	Male	Female
Britain (base rate)	100	100	100	100	100	100	100	100
West Indies	103	113	72a	– 22a }	156d	185d*	136*	156*
Africa			88	59a }			121b	129b
India	85	79			236c*	325c*	149*	123*
Pakistan	68	68	134	191*			59*	55

Notes

There are substantial differences in the rates quoted by different authors for the British-born patients in their series. Presumably these reflect differences in the organization and utilization of psychiatric services in different areas. To obtain rough comparability therefore the rates for each immigrant group have been converted to a percentage of the rates given for British-born patients in the same sample.

* indicates statistically significant difference from British-born rate (p < 0.01) calculated by the authors in each case.

a Hitch comments that the numbers in these categories were too small for any important conclusions to be drawn.

b includes ethnic Africans and ethnic Indians (refugees from Kenya and Uganda).

c all Asians amalgamated, including Bangla Deshis.

d includes 'negroes from sub-Saharan Africa' (13 per cent of sample).

non-patients in having 'higher levels of goal striving,' i.e. they were ambitious. It may be that West Indians find themselves blocked, despite all efforts to improve their conditions, and become frustrated (Bagley 1971b; Schlicht and Carmichael 1976). Several researchers have tried to relate morbidity and duration of stay in Britain, but the results are inconclusive (Cochrane 1977, Joseph 1978). Hill (1975) suggests that immigrants become more neurotic the longer they remain (see below). Ødegaard's Scandinavian figures demonstrate that rural to urban migration is more likely to produce psychiatric problems than rural-to-rural or urban-to-urban migration (Ødegaard 1945; Astrup and Ødegaard 1960). Since the majority of New Commonwealth immigrants are from rural backgrounds, this should be a factor predisposing to high rates. Several writers have commented on the protective value of the 'ethnic enclave' within which people can live and adjust at their own rate. It would be interesting to know the morbidity rates among immigrants who are, and are not, living in such enclaves. Hitch (1975) collected this data for Bradford Asians but could not discern any consistent trends: perhaps because those who move out from the the inner-city wards are the most successful and adaptable. As a rule, admission rates tend to be higher among the less educated, but one study in Canada found that among immigrants from some countries, the rates were higher from the better-educated, perhaps because immigrants who come from very poor conditions are relatively easily satisfied, while the better educated come seeking something more than basic material security, and may find it unattainable (Murphy 1969b).

DIFFERENCES IN PARTICULAR DIAGNOSES

In most of the studies quoted, the statistics seem to show a high incidence of schizophrenia and paranoid psychoses in the immigrant groups (compensated in some groups by a low incidence of affective disorders and neuroses). Because of all the diagnostic pitfalls already described, we can view these figures with some scepticism. It is impossible, of course, to quantify the degree of misdiagnosis but a few pointers are available. Hollingshead and Redlich (1958) pointed out that in social classes I and II about 65 per cent of patients were diagnosed as neurotic, but the percentage decreased down the socio-economic scale to 10 per cent in class V. The figures for schizophrenia are roughly converse. This may be because of a tendency for members of classes I/II to consult psychiatrists about problems that members of other social classes would tackle in some other way, coupled with a tendency for schizophrenics to drift down the social scale. As well as that, however, it seems likely that doctors can more easily understand the problems presented to them by members of social classes I and II because they are more articulate, and because this is the class to which the doctor himself belongs. Incomprehensibility is a factor in the diagnosis of psychosis as against neurosis, and social distance reduces understanding. This is presumably even more true of cultural distance. Tewfik and Okasha (1965) studied 124 West Indian immigrants admitted to hospital and found that although schizophrenia was a common diagnostic label, only 15 per cent of the sample conformed to the classic description of either schizophrenia or manic/depressive psychosis — the remaining 85 per cent had atypical features which made the diagnostic label somewhat imprecise. The so-called 'West Indian Psychosis' may sometimes be classified as schizophrenia, but in Hemsi's view (1967) it 'derives in an understandable fashion from a primary affective change'. Chandrasena, in a retrospective review of twenty-one West Indian and West African so-called 'schizophrenics' in London, found that one-third of them showed none of Schneider's First Rank symptoms (Chandrasena 1979). Dean and his colleagues comment that 'acute psychotic episodes often seen in developing countries' are misleading, and being 'relatively uncommon for contemporary British psychiatrists, may be more likely to be labelled schizophrenia by them' (Dean *et al.* 1981). Carpenter and Brockington (1980) found many immigrants with delusions of persecution but without other features of schizophrenia, and suggested that they be classified as 'paranoid psychosis'. Joseph (1978) noted that the diagnosis given initially to Asian patients was often revised during a period of in-patient observation.

COMMUNITY SURVEYS

Hospital data can only indicate the tip of the iceberg of psychiatric morbidity, and knowing the reluctance of Asians in particular to accept hospitalization, we might suppose that the concealed portion of the iceberg would be very large indeed. This may well be the case, (though the distinction between adaptation problems, unhappiness, and minor mental illness is a difficult one); but oddly enough such data as is available does not suggest it. Cochrane and his colleagues conducted two surveys using the Langner twenty-two-item questionnaire as a measure of psychological disturbance, having first checked its validity on an Asian sample. Their surveys contained altogether 300 Indian and Pakistani respondents (with no psychiatric histories), and they found *less* psychological disturbance among them than among an indigenous comparison group (Cochrane, Hashmi, and Stopes-Roe 1977; Cochrane and Stopes-Roe 1977, 1981; Cochrane 1980). Rutter and his colleagues have studied the children of immigrants (Rutter *et al.* 1974a, 1974b), using a questionnaire designed to discover behavioural disturbance. In a comparison of 100 children of West Indian parents and 250 children of indigenous parents they found only slight and inconsistent differences, and concluded that 'much of the concern about high rates of "problem behaviour" is unjustified'. This relative optimism contrasts with the gloomy picture of 'inadequate West Indian parenting' painted by several previous writers (Price 1967) and with various accounts of ethnic identity crises among black adolescents (Weinreich 1975, 1977; 1979; see also Bagley 1976).

Cochrane used the Rutter questionnaire on a mixed sample of English, West Indian, and Pakistani children in Birmingham. He too found no greater behavioural deviancy among the children of West Indian parents than those of indigenous parents (though in this series they did show a higher incidence of psychiatric hospital admissions). Among the children of Pakistani parents he found a lower rate of deviancy (and psychiatric admission) than among the children of indigenous parents (Cochrane 1979).

Indirect support for these findings comes from the work of Hill (1975) who tested 700 schoolchildren with the Eysenck Junior Personality Inventory and analysed the results by ethnic origin. He found that on the 'Neuroticism' scale, West Indian boys scored marginally higher, and West Indian girls slightly lower, than their English counterparts, but the differences were not statistically significant. Asian children were markedly less neurotic on this scale, the difference between English/West Indian on the one hand and Asian on the other being statistically significant (combined sexes). Neuroticism scores tended to be higher in those who had been longest in Britain.

EXPLANATIONS FOR DIFFERENT RATES

If these are any significant differences in the prevalence of mental illness among different ethnic groups, and if they cannot be entirely attributed to artefact or diagnostic confusion, what other explanations should be considered? Classically there are three theoretical possibilities:

(1) The processes of migration and adjustment are such that they induce mental disorder at a higher (or lower) rate.

(2) The decision to migrate is taken by people who have certain personal characteristics which render them more (or less) liable to mental disorder.

(3) The population of the country of origin has a higher (or lower) morbidity rate, and the migrating group is a representative sample which simply reflects this difference. (Murphy 1977)

Any or all of these factors may apply. Factor (1) may well be the most important in situations of extreme cultural and social deprivation, including the enforced migration of refugees, but even among refugees there is some evidence in favour of (2). Factor (3) is often overlooked, and in respect of immigrants to Britain there is, at present, little prospect of obtaining the data from countries of origin which would throw light on it. Even in a country with a relatively well-developed psychiatric service, such as Barbados, social factors and attitudes to hospitalization combine to produce a pattern of apparent morbidity which is very different from the pattern in Britain. In most parts of the Caribbean, the Indian subcontinent, and Africa, the case-finding services that are a prerequisite of epidemiology simply do not exist.

Kessel has questioned the value of international comparisons at the present time (Kessel 1965). The present author's own view is that quantitative comparisons are beset by so many artefacts, and are so much open to misinterpretation, that research time and resources are better spent on elucidating qualitative differences.

Treatment

Cultural Differences in Attitude to Psychiatric Treatment

FEAR AND STIGMA

Mental disorder commonly evokes fear. Unexpected or peculiar behaviour seems to be inherently alarming, probably because routine human interactions depend on the tacit assumption that our perceptions of the world are all roughly similar and our reactions moderately predictable. If, when you see a rabbit, I see a tiger and run screaming, you experience a sense of shock — all the more so if, up to then, we had both seemed to perceive the same rabbit. To the layman, 'mad' people are frightening because 'you never know what they'll do next', and this perplexity leads to anxious fantasies. Mentally abnormal people are perceived as dangerous.

Anyone with experience of a British psychiatric hospital knows that the vast majority of patients have no particular propensity to violence. There is less risk of being attacked in a mental hospital than in a pub at closing time, yet still the general public equates mental illness with unpredictability, and unpredictability with dangerousness. The same is true in other countries, and sometimes with more reason, since in many cultures violence is an essential criterion of mental illness. In most of Asia, Africa, and the Caribbean, no-one goes to a psychiatrist unless they are 'mad', and no-one is designated 'mad' unless they are violent. A person who is mentally disturbed but not violent is not 'mad'.

This link between violence and madness affects the nature of mental hospitals. With few exceptions, mental hospitals in the Third World are fairly dreadful places, and there are many in which custodial care is the only intention, ECT the usual treatment, staff brutality is commonplace, all patients are compulsorily detained, and few are ever discharged. Where this description is no longer true, it probably *was* true within living memory. Mental hospitals are places of last resort.

Not surprisingly, immigrants from countries to which this applies are likely to view British mental hospitals with trepidation, and equate psychiatry with punishment. 'Why must I go to the mental hospital? I've done nothing wrong!' is a common reaction. A different kind of fear may be met in refugees from totalitarian regimes where the medical profession — psychiatry included — is not guiltless in the matter of torture and political 'rehabilitation'. Others may see psychiatry as an instrument of oppression of blacks by whites.

This last accusation is not as bizarre as first appears. Wherever a colonial administration has the task of 'keeping the natives in order' there are two sanctions that can be supplied to really troublesome dissidents — they can be locked up in prison if they are sane, or in a mental hospital if mad. In (for example) Jamaica before independence, nearly every patient admitted to Bellevue Hospital was sent from court, having been found guilty of some kind of socially unacceptable (probably violent) behaviour. The atmosphere was more penal than therapeutic. In other colonies the mental hospital might be under the same administration as the prison, even an annexe to it. Bearing in mind all the diagnostic pitfalls already listed, we may reasonably suppose that the judicial establishment (white) sometimes erred in distinguishing between mad violence and sane violence, and despatched the socially undesirable (black) to the wrong institution. Going back a little further in history we find the diagnosis of 'Drapetomania' being applied to American slaves who exhibited the 'pathological' symptom of wishing to be free (Littlewood and Lipsedge 1982). Even today, there is evidence of political abuse of psychiatry in the maintenance of apartheid in South Africa (WHO 1977; Sashidharan 1981). While such suspicions linger, British psychiatrists cannot expect automatic immunity from them.

Mental disorder also induces shame, in the family as well as the sufferer. In even the most enlightened societies it is probably easier to admit: 'My son has leukaemia' than: 'My daughter has anorexia nervosa'. This shame has at least two roots: on the one hand people might suspect that my daughter is ill because she has been mishandled, psychologically traumatized; mental disorder suggests failings in upbringing. On the other hand, there is the common belief that 'insanity runs in families' — i.e. it has a genetic component. Both explanations contain a germ of truth, which keeps them alive. The genetic argument in particular appeals to people whose background is agricultural, since they know about the existence of inherited characteristics. Desirable attributes can be encouraged in farm animals by selective breeding, so presumably the same is true of human beings. It is natural to assume that an affliction which has no other obvious cause is 'in the blood'. In cultures in which marriages are arranged by elders, great care is taken to establish the respectability of bride and groom, and of their antecedents. If it were known that there is a 'streak of insanity' in a family, this would affect marriage prospects for other members as well as the patient. Stigmatization may make the family prefer concealment to treatment.

CAUSES OF MENTAL ILLNESS

Clarke (1979) has reported a study in which Barbadians in Barbados and in Britain were asked what they thought were the causes of madness. Among those mentioned were:

(1) *'Studiation'* (as in 'He's been studying too much'). This does not necessarily refer to academic endeavour. To study is to think intently or reflect about an issue (an old English usage which persists also in northern English dialect). The idea that one can damage one's mind by mental over-exertion is persuasive, and crops up elsewhere in the diagnosis of 'Brain Fag Syndrome' used by some African psychiatrists.

(2) *'People can make you mad'*. Two mechanisms were suggested: (a) tampering with food or drink, and (b) Obeah. Obeah is the general Caribbean term for witchcraft and magic. The Obeah Man or Obeah Women has mysterious powers which can be used for good or evil purposes. Like witchcraft in Britain, Obeah encompasses elements of perverted Christianity, animism, folk-medicine and herbal toxicology, superstition, and personal malevolence. The 'Wise Woman' who has healing powers based on traditional remedies, is also credited with the power to do harm. To 'put an Obeah on' a person might involve (for example) obtaining bones from a cemetery and placing them in the victim's path.

(3) *'Taking things on'* (or *'Letting things get to you'*). These phrases presumably include failing to keep a sense of proportion, brooding, or failing to rise above some misfortune.

(4) *Insufficient period of rest after childbirth*. The belief is that it takes time for the body to knit together again. A midwife who tries to mobilize her patient in the puerperium may encounter this objection.

(5) *High blood pressure associated with being in the hot sun*.

(6) *Inheritance* – 'Bad blood' (see above).

Clarke states that the vernacular expression for bewitched is 'foolish'. The term 'madness' is reserved for people who are not only 'foolish' but also violent. However, some flexibility is allowed – a member of one's own family or village is more likely to be described as 'foolish', an outsider as 'mad'. An eccentric or feeble-minded person might be termed 'an idiot', but not 'mad'. To be depressed, however severely, is not madness either.

Among Indians and Pakistanis, magical and supernatural explanations are often put forward, and examples of these have been given in Chapters 12 and 20. Other factors include inheritance (see above); deliberate poisoning by an enemy; unbalanced diet; climate; immoral behaviour (including sexual excess or malpractice). Muslims may simply refer to 'The Will of Allah' and derive comfort from that belief. This may help — but occasionally it may hinder, since one cannot object to or get angry about that which is Allah's will, so that legitimate expression of emotion is sometimes prevented when it might be therapeutic. The fatalism of Hinduism is somewhat different, and includes the concepts of *Karma* and *Dharma*, which relate to preordained patterns of behaviour connected with actions in previous incarnations. The influence of the stars may be another factor. Any mental abnormality in a young unmarried man or woman may be attributed indirectly to sex: the association may not be mentioned directly, but the suggestion is often made that marriage would solve the problem. In Chinese and Vietnamese cultures, ghosts play a large part in human affairs, and a person who experiences feelings of apprehension, anxiety, or depression may assume that their house is haunted.

Among all these ascribed causes, some are more socially acceptable than others, and the degree of stigma varies accordingly. In societies in which science, medicine, philosophy, and religion are not separated into different compartments, there is not the same distinction between factual explanation and moral judgement. A British practitioner may describe an illness as 'bad', but shrink from describing the patient as 'bad'. We say that there is 'something wrong with' a person, without meaning to imply that the patient has done wrong. Moral issues are not our province, but this dichotomy only makes sense in a science-based society, and is not immediately obvious to others. In European cultures there are experts in physical health, mental health, spiritual health, social policy, and so on. They are different 'subjects'. In Eastern thought: 'There is a strong belief that all events have a place within a supernatural logic' (Ballard 1979 : 156). There are unseen forces at work, and any unexplained affliction (especially anything sinister like madness) gives rise to the suspicion that its victim is an unfortunate person — not merely in the sense that his illness is a misfortune, but with a deeper apprehension that fortune (or something) is not on his side. It is prudent to avoid becoming too closely involved with such a person, or with his family.

PHENOMENOLOGY, DIAGNOSIS, AND ASKING THE WRONG QUESTIONS

The British practitioner has been trained in the 'Sherlock Holmes' diagnostic method. By obtaining an accurate description of the symptoms and signs, and their mode of development, and examining the patient, he aims to build up a picture of the type of condition he is dealing with. He wants to know 'what?' before he starts to ask 'why?'. But for many patients these phenomenological questions seem to be the wrong questions. In the eyes of many Asian patients (and probably others), the doctor ought to know *what* is wrong without asking questions: the patient already knows *what* is wrong, he has come to the doctor to find out *why*. Methodical working through a phenomenological check-list does not instil confidence, it undermines it. This distinction between 'what' and 'why' questions depends on the acceptance of disease entities. For example, after examining a patient who has a cough, a doctor might say that the cough is due to bronchitis, and that he will treat the bronchitis, whereupon the cough will disappear. If pressed, he will explain that he is not giving treatment for the cough, but for the underlying bronchitis. If further pressed he will say that he does not know why the patient has contracted bronchitis — but the question is irrelevant. This all makes sense to a person who has some conception of the existence of an entity called 'bronchitis' which he has 'got'. If, however, there is no such concept of a disease entity, all that the patient hears the doctor say is that he is giving some treatment which will eventually relieve the cough, and he does not know what has caused it: which does not sound very impressive.

In this case the doctor could (if permitted) justify his use of the term 'bronchitis' by reference to demonstrable pathological changes in the chest. The psychiatrist is in a more difficult position. He can say that the hallucinations are due to schizophrenia and that he is treating the underlying condition, but he cannot so easily demonstrate that schizophrenia exists as an entity. His admission that he does not know why the patient has developed the illness destroys any vestige of credibility. In the eyes of a patient (or relative) who does not subscribe to the 'disease-entity' concept, he is providing symptom relief only, and not even attempting to tackle the roots of the problem. The questions he ought to be asking, and the advice he ought to be giving, are in terms of the ascribed causes, some of which are mentioned above. The patient is not asking 'What have I got?' but possibly 'Who did it?' or 'Where am I going wrong? The question 'Why is my wife ill?' may really mean 'Why did it have to be my wife — not someone else?' or even 'Why does God permit the existence of suffering?' — questions that most British patients do not ask, and which few British doctors are prepared to tackle.

It would help if we could identify particular syndromes that are likely to have, in the patient's view, particular causes. If, for example, auditory hallucinations are usually a sign of divine or supernatural intervention, while somatic discomfort are usually attributable to human enmity, manic over-activity to astrological forces, and so on. This is not (as far as we are aware) the case in any of the cultures under discussion here. Causes and effects are not correlated in that way. It is not suggested that when the patient or the patient's relatives attribute illness to particular causes (e.g. magic) the practitioner should necessarily play along with them and pretend to beliefs which he does not hold. This question is considered in some detail in Chapter 20. The point relevant here is simply that the questions of precise phenomenology beloved of Western diagnosticians do not fit into the conceptual models used in other cultures, and by asking these questions (essential though they are) the doctor may be losing credibility, since he is revealing ignorance rather than wisdom and failing to address fundamental causes. However the causes may be envisaged, it is hard for the patient to believe that pills alone will negate them. Up to a point, this is an attitude that many psychiatrists would applaud. Where the disorder is due to stress and conflict, be it internal or interpersonal, we might well agree that pills are not the answer, and wish to engage in some form of psychotherapy with a view to the modification of attitudes and habitual behaviour. The psychiatrist, more than most other doctors, should be willing to take into account all aspects of his patient's life situation, and to adopt a perspective which goes beyond the narrowly 'medical' model. The social caseworker will certainly wish to do so. It would seem, therefore, that these professions ought to come closer to the ideal of the 'healer' as it is construed in other (e.g. Asian) cultures. Paradoxically, this does not work out in practice. A psychiatrist who attempts to work psychotherapeutically with an Asian patient may well get the response, at the end of the session: 'Thank you for the talk, doctor, it was very interesting: but aren't you going to prescribe me some treatment?' (noted by Bavington (1981, personal communication)). Two reasons for this may be suggested. One is to do with the doctor's allotted role: he is perceived as a person who dispenses drugs and that is what he is expected to do. Other sorts of healers may have more to offer (see next chapter): what British doctors have is drugs, injections, X-rays, and technological gadgets. They may be of limited value, but they are not available elsewhere, and they are the reason for consulting him — even if he is to be criticized at the same time for his limited view.

In some situations this attitude works to advantage. Asian patients maintained on depot phenothiazines are (in the author's experience) very reliable in turning up regularly. The idea of coming to the clinic once every month to have an injection which will prevent them getting sick again, fits very well the conceptual model (though occasionally a patient may announce that he will not be needing to come any more since he has now solved the problem (having perhaps been to Mecca, or got married). Long-term pill-taking is not so impressive, and compliance is much less. If medication is regarded as symptom-relief only, it follows that drugs which do not relieve symptoms quickly are no good, and are not likely to be persisted with — a problem with antidepressants in particular.

PSYCHOTHERAPY

Another reason why non-drug approaches to treatment are often ineffective may have something to do with the techniques that the psychotherapist (or caseworker) adopts. A British therapist probably sees himself or herself as an *enabler*. By helping the patient to see for himself what is happening, by bringing into conscious awareness some factors which were influencing the patient without his knowledge, the patient is *enabled* to make choices for himself. By being non-judgemental the therapist enables the patient to express and explore his own feelings, and by being non-directive he obliges the patient to make his own decisions. Psychotherapy of this kind may suit some highly educated subjects in individualistic and introspective societies, but it cannot be applied everywhere. In most traditional societies if you do not know what to do you go to a wise man and ask him, and he tells you. You might not always follow his advice, but at least you expect him to give it, not bounce the question back at you. So it is with the healer: he is expected to give detailed and precise instructions (which may include instructions on several different aspects of living). It is not necessary for the patient to understand why he has to carry them out (though they must fit in somehow to the patient's belief-systems). The British doctor who adopts the 'I'm-not-going-to-tell-you-what-to-do-let's-see-if-we-can-work-it-out-together' approach may leave the patient unsatisfied and bewildered. Even within British or American culture, psychotherapy is affected by differences in attitude and expectation due to social class and educational background:

> 'All too often, psychotherapy runs into difficulties when the therapist and the patient belong to different classes. The most frequent source of difficulty . . . is the patient's overt or tacit demand for an authoritarian attitude on the part of the psychiatrist, and the psychiatrist's unwillingness to assume this role because it runs counter to certain therapeutic principles. "Insight" therapy is less likely to be grasped by lower class patients than physical therapy or a therapy employing "magical" methods.'   (Hollingshead and Redlich 1958 : 345)

The same difficulties arise across cultural, as well as social, boundaries. In patients from Asian cultures we may also discern some conceptual difficulties arising from different concepts of the self. This has already been discussed in Chapters 10 and 12. Where introspection is not encouraged, and a person's identity is much more bound up with relationships and roles than with purely subjective experience, self-analysis in the post-Freudian mode may seem a strange and difficult undertaking. The 'self-regarding ego' which is an essential participant in the process of analytic or introspective psychotherapy does not seem to be available.

Transference phenomena are likely to be problematic whenever the cultural backgrounds of therapist and patient are very dissimilar. The therapist may suspect that he is enacting the role of father-figure in the patient's emotional life, but may discover that an Indian or Afro-Caribbean father-figure is somewhat different from a British one. Even if we abandon strict Freudian concepts, the need for rapport and empathy remains, and these are most easily established when the two participants have life experiences and value systems in common. Para-phrasing the Inverse Square Law of Physics, we may say that empathy diminishes as the square of the cultural distance.

Another way of looking at what happens in psychotherapy is to regard the interaction within the session as a paradigm for interactions that occur in 'real life' outside. A therapist might say: 'Let us stop and analyse the conversation we have just had . . . look at the way you are behaving towards me, now, in this situation . . . the way you feel about me at the moment . . . because maybe that's the way you behave towards other people, the way you feel about other people, outside?' The patient may be emboldened to express some 'dangerous' feelings or try out some new experimental modes of interaction, because the therapy situation is hedged round with safeguards and is not 'for real'. Such an approach is obviously culture-bound, and quite alien to anyone whose relationships (and feelings about them) are predetermined by social structure and duty.

FAMILY THERAPY

The classical techniques of psychotherapy that focus on the individual — his or her own experiences and feelings, what happens inside his or her own head — may be difficult to apply in some other cultures, but these techniques are not all that popular in Britain anyway. Increasingly therapists and caseworkers have started to pay more attention to the interpersonal than to the intrapersonal, and have developed techniques of group therapy and family therapy in which there is exploration of interactions. Having described some of the cultures of ethnic minorities in Britain as family-centred, we might think that these approaches would be particularly appropriate for them. So they might, but some modifications will be required, and perhaps we have not yet learned how to make them. Farrar (a social worker with considerable experience of Pakistani clients) states:

'As the client will be in negotiation with other family members about decisions he must make, or particular course of action he must take, it is worthwhile recognizing this and working with it rather than ignoring it or seeing it as a "complication".' Family discussions are part of the client's everyday life, and can be usefully used.

However, rigidity of roles, and the fact that there is a definite hierarchy within the family has also to be recognised. Thus the idea that a wife could openly show her negative feelings towards her husband with a stranger present is almost incomprehensible, and can be seen as very damaging. Expressions of difficulty have to be made through "normal channels" (for example, a wife who is having difficulty with her husband may well talk to her husband's mother about this in the first instance). Allowing difficulties within the family to be seen by other people is damaging to the status of the family itself, and great efforts are made by the family concerned not to let this happen. A social worker therefore has to be accepted almost as a family member, and certainly his ability to retain confidentiality has to be believed before he can work effectively in this way.'

(Farrar 1981 : 8)

Throughout this section there have been generalizations made about 'Asian' or 'West Indian' or other cultural modes of thought: these are, of course, stereotypes, useful only as long as their limitations are kept firmly in mind.

Alternative Medicine

Every society has professional healers, and it is no surprise that any substantial group of immigrants brings with it the system of medicine to which it is accustomed. Thus, alongside orthodox medical services, we have a whole variety of culture-bound alternative medical systems. *Tavees* are readily obtainable in the Muslim community in Britain, Tiger Balm can be purchased in any city, a person troubled by evil spirits need not look far to find an exorcist.

'Alternative medicine' has long flourished in Britain, and it includes homeopathy, herbalism, osteopathy and chiropractice, spiritualism and hypnotherapy. Their appeal is not diminishing, and the addition of newly imported techniques is a variation on an existing theme. Alternative medicine exists in parallel with the National Health Service; like parallel lines, they never meet.

Only one of the alternative medical services used by ethnic minorities has been subjected to any systematic research, and that is the practice of *Unani* medicine in the Pakistani community. An extensive study of these systems and their practitioners, the *Hakims* and *Vaids*, has been undertaken in the last five years by Dr Mohammad Aslam and his colleagues and has yielded some unexpected discoveries. In this chapter we shall attempt to summarize some of Aslam's findings with particular reference to mental illness.[1] Aslam had the advantage of being an Urdu-speaker familiar with Pakistani culture and medical beliefs, at the same time as being a British-trained pharmacist with access to research facilities and analytical techniques. In the course of his study he was able to be present with several Hakims while they saw patients and discuss with them the diagnosis and treatment of a series of cases. He was able to obtain samples of the drugs prescribed for chemical and pharmacological analysis. He also sat in at psychiatric clinics, and was able to make direct comparisons of the techniques used by both types of practitioners about similar cases (including, on a few occasions, the same patient).

HAKIMS AND VAIDS

Hakims are practitioners of the *Unani* (or *Unani-Tibb*) systems of medicine utilized throughout the Islamic world. Unani is a development of Arab traditional medicine and has common ancestry with European medicine as far back as Galen and Hippocrates. In fact, many of the concepts of Unani medicine are vaguely familiar to British doctors who have attended lectures on the history of medicine. According to Unani medicine, there are four main humours in the body, namely blood, phlegm, yellow bile, and black bile, and these must be kept in balance if health is to be maintained. They have the characteristics of being either 'hot' or 'cold' and either 'wet' or 'dry'. Thus blood is both hot and wet, yellow bile is dry and hot, and so on. A particular illness may be due to an excess of heat or cold, wetness or dryness in the body, and treatment consists of restoring the balance. Within limits people differ in their normal make-up, and can thus be characterized as sanguine (if blood predominates), phlegmatic (phlegm), melancholic (yellow bile), or choleric (black bile).

Vaids, or Vaidya, are practitioners of *Ayurvedic* medicine which is the traditional medicine of India and derives ultimately from Hindu beliefs. In Ayurveda there are three natural 'elements'; wind, water, and fire, and these are represented in the body by three humours; namely breath, phlegm, and bile. Once again, health depends on the proper balance of these three, illness is characterized by an excess or deficiency of one or other, and treatment is directed at correcting this.

The differences between Unani and Ayurvedic medicine have been eroded by time. Between them, they provide about 65 per cent of the medical services in India and Pakistan. Properly speaking a practitioner in those countries may not call himself a Hakim or Vaid unless he has undergone a course of training which is comparable in length and complexity to the medical training in Britain. There are Unani and Ayurvedic medical colleges and hospitals, in which every type of condition is treated by traditional methods, either alone or in conjunction with imported European remedies, and a massive pharmaceutical industry (The Hamdard Foundation) comparable in scale to Messrs Boots in Britain (see also Dastur 1960). In the villages, a local healer who has no formal training but has knowledge of herbal remedies, may be referred to as a Hakim, and he is often the only medical practitioner of any kind in the neighbourhood. Qualified or not, the Hakim is the usual source of treatment once the resources of the household have been tried and failed. It is not surprising that when Aslam carried out a questionnaire survey of a sample of Asians in Britain, 232 out of 250 respondents stated that they had consulted Hakims in the past in India or Pakistan. An unexpected finding was that 202 out of 250 still consulted Hakims in Britain.

THE PRACTICE OF A RESIDENT HAKIM IN BRITAIN

During four weeks spent in the surgery of a resident full-time Hakim in a British city, Aslam watched the diagnosis and treatment of seventy-nine patients and among these the diagnosis (made by the Hakim) included:

Psychosexual problems	22
Undue tiredness	10
Nerves, depression, irritability	2
Palpitations	2
	36

(The other major diagnostic group was digestive problems (nineteen cases).) It appears that about half the cases had (in the Hakim's opinion) some complaint which might be regarded as psychiatric, and it is likely that psychosomatic factors entered into some of the others. Aslam himself states 'The majority of the cases which come to a Hakim involve psychiatric problems' (Aslam 1979 : 241).

How were the diagnoses made? Mainly, it seemed, on the state of the pulse, which the Hakim felt at the wrist, using two fingers:

'The beat generally felt by the forefinger gives some indication of the state of the humours. To learn whether bile is involved in the trouble, the middle finger is used. The ring finger can determine whether all is well with phlegm. Because of assumed differences in the circulatory systems of the sexes, the Hakim used the right hand of the male patient for examination and the left hand of the female. He claims to be able to diagnose up to twenty ailments by this method.'   (Aslam 1979 : 78)

The diagnostic importance of the pulse was mentioned in earlier (Indian) reports (Carstairs 1958a). No other form of physical examination was considered necessary. However, this is plainly not the whole story. The Hakim spent time listening to the patient as well.

'Within the Western communities a patient visiting the local physician will relate the symptoms of his or her affliction and be prescribed a remedy . . . on average the patient spends about five minutes in consultation with the doctor. In contrast the Asian healer (Hakim or Vaid) will spend a much longer time with his patient in getting to know him or her and in providing a counselling service.'
                                                  (Aslam 1979 : 12)

Local knowledge, understanding the culture of his particular local clientele, seemed to Aslam to be the main (and important) asset of the local Hakim. 'He is greatly respected and his advice is sought on many matters of both health and welfare in the community' (Aslam 1979 : 96).

THE VISITING HAKIM

'Two weeks prior to the Hakim's arrival . . . notices were sent out by his representative in London to each of his previous patients . . . Then during this fortnight various notices made their appearance in grocery and drapery stores . . . giving the full address where the clinic was to be held and the dates and times . . . Similar advertisements were placed in Asian newspapers, including a photograph of the Hakim.'
(Aslam 1979 : 112)

Aslam spent four days with this visiting Hakim who had set up a clinic in a London hotel and kept records of ninety-six patients: 49 per cent travelled from outside London, some from as far as Scotland, Tyneside, and West Yorkshire. One had even come from Holland. Seventy-five per cent were men, predominantly in the age group 25–44 years. Many had consulted him on a previous visit. The Hakim had his own system of classification, according to which the following diagnoses were recorded:

Infective	8	Nutritional	14
Mental	26	Circulatory	14
Digestive	9	Genito-Urinary	8
Skin	5	Musculoskeletal	8
Others	4		

Once again, it seems that psychiatric or psychosomatic conditions form a large part of the Hakim's practice, and of these, a substantial proportion were partly if not entirely psychosexual problems. Again it seemed that the main therapeutic asset was the time and understanding given to the patient, reinforced in this case by the prestige of the 'visiting consultant' image.

TREATMENT

In accordance with the basic principals of Unani or Ayurvedic medicine, treatment depends on restoring the body's balance in terms of 'hot' and 'cold' humours. Some conditions can be picked out as due to excess heat or cold, and Aslam quotes the following examples:

Heat	Cold
Pregnancy	Lactation
Skin rashes and irritations	Paralysis or stiffness of any part of
Kidney pains	the body; rheumatism
Toothache (molars)	Pain in front teeth, teething in infants
Dysentery	Diarrhoea of other types

A 'hot' condition may be attributed to eating too much 'hot' food, but whether it has been caused by faulty diet or not, correct diet usually plays a large part in treatment. Particular foods are regarded as either hot or cold and either wet or dry: this bears no relationship to the temperature, nor does it reflect spiciness: in fact, to Western eyes there seems to be no logic in the classification, as the following table (adapted from Aslam 1979) indicates.

Examples of 'hot' and 'cold' foods

Hot	Cold
All meat and fish	
Carrots, aubergines, lettuce, onions, peas, peppers, tomatoes	Cabbage, cauliflower, cucumbers, *bhindi*, potatoes, pumpkins, spinach
Apples*, bananas, grapes*, mangoes,* melons, olives	Citrus fruits, peaches, pears, pineapples, plums, lychees, watermelon
Most nuts, currents, raisins, dates, figs	
Millet, sago, most pulses	Barley, maize, rice
Butter, oil	Cheese, yoghurt
Sugar, honey	Vinegar
Tea	
Most spices except coriander	Egg white

(* except when sour or unripe, when they are 'cold')

Aslam notes that pregnancy is a 'hot' condition, and therefore in pregnancy one should not eat many 'hot' foods, but as the above list shows, most of the protein-rich foods are in the 'hot' category. Aslam interviewed seventy-nine Asian pregnant women in Bradford and found that 59 per cent of them held strongly to these dietary beliefs. Is this, perhaps, a factor in the low birth-weights commonly noted in Asian babies? In addition to advice on diet, the Hakim might give advice on other aspects of living.

'The philosophy of the (Unani) system is that by conserving symmetry in the different spheres of a man's life, the man's health will be

protected. Hence the task of the practitioner . . . became not so
much how to cure the patient as to teach the patient how to con-
serve or restore his own symmetry.'   (Aslam 1979 : 44)

Every patient would receive a prescription, usually made up specially
for the individual by the Hakim in his own dispensary. A typical remedy
might contain products of sixteen different herbs and a dozen or more
other additives. The Indian equivalent of the National Formulary is the
Hamdard Pharmacopeia, which gives the 'standard' recipes for a long
list of named products recommended for particular conditions. Aslam
found, however, that the medicines manufactured and prescribed by
local Hakims in Britain often differed very considerably from the
standard preparation, and a Hakim would be able to defend this on the
grounds that he was producing a remedy specific to the needs of ths
individual.

How effective are these remedies? Aslam found that two-thirds of
the patients who consult Hakims are satisfied with the treatment they
receive, and believe that it is of benefit to them: but this does not mean
that the medication itself is therapeutic. It may be, or it may not be.
We do know that certain plant extracts have pharmacological actions.
Opium, cannabis and digitalis are obvious examples, but the list of
substances which originally came into medicine from herbalists includes
also atropine, colchicine, codeine, coumarin, ephedrine, hyoscine,
nicotine, papaverine, quinidine, quinine, reserpine, strychinine, and
theophylline. It is likely that some of the herbs used by Hakims have
biological activity, just as some of the 'old wives' tales' about onion,
garlic, and other indigenous plants may yet be scientifically vindicated.
Aslam analysed samples of several preparations used by Hakims in
Britain. He found several harmless substances such as cane sugar,
potassium carbonate, sodium borate, and iron, and also several substances known to have pharmacological activity including aconite, nux
vomica, naphthaquinone, and a variety of alkaloids and glycosides. He
also found, in a good many of the preparations, significant quantities
of mercury, tin, gold, lead, and arsenic; and it is these metals, which
are known to be toxic, which give definite grounds for alarm about the
Hakim's medicines.

One group of medicines which must be regarded as definitely
dangerous are the *Kushtay* which are commonly prescribed for chronic
illness but particularly as aphrodisiacs (for both sexes).

'Hakims have been much more ready than their western counterparts
to recognise that many Asians are very anxious about their psychosexual problems and have been prepared to offer some sort of
remedy. All the Hakims seem to prescribe these remedies which are

regarded as a perfectly respectable part of their considerable medical
armamentarium and they are known as Kushtay. All are taken
internally by males and females . . . Their composition is mainly
oxidised heavy metals such as lead, mercury, silver, gold, arsenic
and zinc.'   (Aslam 1979 : 357)

Most British Hakims manufacture Kushtay to their own specifications.
Some are sold 'over the counter' or by post. It is also possible for a
patient to purchase from the Hakim the individual ingredients and
manufacture his own — a particularly hazardous practice.

Bal Jivan Chamcho is a baby tonic, marketed in India as a panacea
for 'Children's diseases, *viz* varadha capilliary, bronchitis, greenish
diarrhoea, rickets, cough, convulsions, etc.'. It has a unique form of
presentation, being hard paste adhering firmly to a teaspoon. The spoon
is stirred into a small amount of warm milk until the colour permeates
the milk, which is then fed to the child off the same spoon. Unfortunately, whatever benefits the paste might have, the teaspoon contains a
very high proportion of lead (43–83 per cent by weight in spoons
analysed by Aslam) which also diffuse into the milk. This 'tonic' therefore produces chronic lead poisoning in the child. Its importation has
now been specifically prohibited under the Medicines Act.

Surma — the grey-black cosmetic used by Asian women as a mascara
— is also a cause of lead poisoning, since many varieties of Surma consist largely of lead sulphide. Aslam and his colleagues have carried out
considerable research in this field, and the dangers of Surma, particularly when used by pregnant women or by children, are becoming
better known. (Ali *et al.* 1978; Aslam *et al.* 1979, 1980; Green *et al.*
1979; Fernando *et al.* 1981). One of the consequences of lead poisoning
is brain damage, so the issue has psychiatric implications: it has been
suggested that the higher incidence of mental handicap noted in some
surveys of Asian children might be due to this factor among others.
Surmas are not merely cosmetic, they are thought to have beneficial
effects on the eye. Special surmas, known as *Kuhl* are manufactured
and prescribed by Hakims. Therapeutic claims include:

Tonic for the eye.
Prophylactic for ocular diseases.
Helps the retention of good eyesight till the advent of old age.
Removes the opacity of the eye, pterygium and xerophthalmia.
Useful in incipient cataract.

(Aslam 1979)

These claims have not been substantiated.
In general, we have to conclude from Aslam's research that what-

ever the merits of the Hakim as an advice-giver and counsellor, the preparations which he prescribes are at best unproven and at worst definitely harmful. Most Asians find this hard to credit. They point out that these traditional remedies have been in use for centuries, and if they had ill-effects that would surely have come to light earlier. There are two reasons why this might not be so. First, in a society that has very high mortality rates through infectious and deficiency diseases, the additional effect of (for example) lead poisoning could easily pass unnoticed. Second, while an official Hakim or Vaid in Pakistan or India is highly trained and may be presumed to have professional competence in his speciality, this is not true of the majority who practice in Britain. Because the qualifications of a Hakim are not recognized in Britain, there is no restriction on anyone laying claim to this title. Most of those who do so would not be permitted to practice in their own country, and some would certainly be regarded as charlatans there.

In addition to the possible toxicity of some of the preparations which he analysed, Aslam points out certain other hazards. A preparation called 'Magsol' is sold extensively at about £12 per jar, and is widely believed to be a cure for gonorrhea. On analysis Aslam found that it consists of a mixture of sugar and sand. Plainly, a person who believes that his gonorrhea has been cured when in fact it has not, remains at risk and may infect others. This is a clear example of the dangers of 'cures' that are not cures. On the other hand, some seemingly innocuous compounds may contain very untraditional constituents, e.g.

'Several materials we have analysed which are available from both resident and visiting Hakims have been found to contain testosterone. For example the product *Neoba* manufactured by Hamdard and prescribed for psychosexual problems.' (Aslam 1979 : 96)

Another risk is that biologically active substances present in traditional medicines, while not in themselves harmful, may interact with other drugs. An example of this is the vegetable *Karela* (which is also used in the preparation of curries) which interacts with chlorpropamide and may produce hypoglycaemia in an otherwise-stabilized diabetic (Aslam and Stockley 1979). Finally, there is at least a strong suspicion that illegal abortions may be carried out by Hakims, using herbal aborti-facients or even (it is alleged) by surgery.

HAKIMS AND PSYCHIATRIC PATIENTS

'(Doctors) must believe, on the whole, what their patients believe, just as they must wear the sort of hat their patients wear ... when the patient has a prejudice the doctor must either keep it in

countenance or lose his patient . . . if he gets ahead of the super-
stitions of his patients he is a ruined man.'

(Shaw, *The Doctor's Dilemma*)

In respect of mental illness, the evidence suggests that Hakims deal
with a great many cases of neurosis and psychosomatic illness, in which
communication and cultural sensitivity are vital, and they offer a specific
service for sexual dysfunction. These are areas in which the British
practitioner has relatively little to offer.

'Hakims are strikingly more acceptable to Asian patients than
Western-style doctors . . . probably related to the readiness of the
Hakim to devote a long time to listening to the patient, and his
invariable readiness to offer advice and medication. Although
patients have to pay for their medicines, they felt they got their
money's worth.'   (Aslam 1979 : 170)

Patients do not consult Hakims *instead* of Western doctors, but *as well
as*. The usual sequence is to consult the general practitioner, then
another doctor privately and/or referral to a hospital specialist, and
then — if still dissatisfied or uncured — consult a Hakim. Hakims are
therefore picking up those cases in which orthodox medicine is perceived to have failed. It is not surprising, therefore, that in Aslam's
sample 60 per cent said they were more satisfied with the Hakim than
the doctor, and only 4 per cent said they had been more satisfied with
the doctor than the Hakim. Even in disorders for which there is no cure,
the Hakim offers hope. In a case of a child with Down's Syndrome
(recorded by Aslam) the mother was so disheartened by the therapeutic
nihilism of British doctors that despite her scepticism she took the child
to an Ayurvedic practitioner. Her scepticism was understandable since
she was herself a general practitioner in Britain. Aware of the underlying nature of the condition, she nonetheless felt that the herbal
remedies which were applied did produce some reduction of the child's
disabilities. At any rate, the fact that something was being done made
her and her husband feel better. Therapeutic optimism is not an unmixed
blessing, however, and Aslam records another case in which two children
with muscular dystrophy were promised a cure by Hakims and priests,
and their parents felt the more disillusioned and depressed when the
cure was not forthcoming.

In many ways the Hakim seems to resemble the English doctor of a
generation ago, whose aim was: 'To cure sometimes, to relieve often,
to comfort always' — and perhaps he achieves this by much the same
methods. If so, there is a lesson here for English doctors of the present
generation, and it is particularly applicable to neuroses, psychosomatic
illness, and conditions on the borderline of mental illness.

In respect of major mental illness — psychosis — the advantage probably lies the other way. There is no evidence that any of the drugs used by Hakims have any therapeutic value (Rauwolfia is an exception, but its disadvantages outweigh its benefits) so perhaps these patients should be left to the psychiatrist. A patient described by Aslam (and with whom the present author was also involved) exemplifies this. He was a forty-five-year old Pakistani from a rural background who had been in Britain for five years but spoke little English, and he complained to his general practitioner of a burning sensation in the stomach, other bodily pains, and voices which he could hear emanating from his chest. He said this was due to one of his workmates who had 'poisoned' his tea by witchcraft. The family was anxious that he should not be labelled as a psychiatric patient. The general practitioner prescribed chlorpromazine, but:

> 'During this period the patient was also attending a visiting Hakim. (He) was advised by the Hakim not to take the chlorpromazine since English medicines were regarded as "hot". It was the view of the Hakim that the patient already had "too much heat", and that the two were clearly contraindicated.'

(This belief that English medicines are all 'hot' is very general, and probably contributes to the poor compliance figures that Aslam and others have reported elsewhere (Aslam, Davis and Fletcher 1979). Since, for example, pregnancy is a hot condition English medicines are considered inappropriate in pregnancy. Since lactation is 'cold' it is clearly absurd to take the same tablets before *and* after childbirth.)

> 'The visiting Hakim diagnosed that the patient's main problem was due to too much heat in the body. The wife of the patient had agreed to obtain the best treatment from the Hakim and paid the maximum fees (£200). The visiting Hakim had assured the family that the patient would be cured. At the same time the patient was also attending a Mullah to obtain some explanation for his illness; in particular why he had been singled out for his illness. He was given some amulets (with curative prayers written from Koran) to wear around his neck. The Mullah said the illness would improve in a few weeks. The cost to the patient was £5.
>
> The relatives of the patient agreed that in their view neither the Hakim's nor the Mullah's treatment had worked. No improvement was found. The patient was then admitted to a psychiatric hospital and was diagnosed as a schizophrenic. After a course of ECT and phenothiazine (he) improved considerably and was discharged from the hospital. In this case despite the greater acceptability of the systems used by the Hakim and Mullah it was the medicine from the psychiatric clinic that eventually proved successful.

In this particular case the patient only admitted to the author (Aslam) about visiting the Hakim and using his medicines. The relatives were well aware of the possible reaction of the general practitioner and the hospital consultant had the patient admitted that he had been to see a Hakim. The main reason given by the patient and his relatives for consulting the Hakim was that they had read in the Asian newspaper of the success of this Hakim and had felt obliged to do the best possible for him.'

(Aslam 1979 : 250–54)

The opposite case, in which the psychiatrist fails and the Hakim succeeds, is probably just as common.

THE FUTURE OF HAKIMS IN BRITAIN – IS COLLABORATION POSSIBLE?

Aslam concludes that the contribution that the Hakims are making to the treatment of illness in the Asian community ought to be recognized and put on an official footing, so that the dangerous or undesirable aspects of their practices can be controlled and the positive therapeutic aspects encouraged. He draws attention to other forms of traditional medicine in Britain that co-exist with orthodox (allopathic) medicine and attract a large and probably increasing clientele. In seems likely, on the face of it, that the legislation that exists to monitor and control the practice of herbalism could be modified to meet the new situation, and if this were done sensitively it would not destroy the position of the Hakim and might even strengthen it. Can we foresee a time when psychiatrist and Hakim could work alongside each other, each referring to the other those patients for whom each was the most appropriate?

This happens in India. The author has been present at a conversation in an Indian village, when the local Hakim had correctly diagnosed a young girl as psychotic, realized that the condition was beyond his competence, and asked the visiting psychiatrist to see her. The two practitioners discussed the case as colleagues, their mutual respect including a certain amount of good-natured banter. The 'Hakim' in this case had no formal training, having learned his skills from his father before him. Nonetheless he was able to give a very clear account of the kinds of nervous complaint he could treat, and as far as an observer could tell his treatments made good therapeutic sense (though the constituents of his medications were not revealed).

It is difficult to envisage such a situation occurring in Britain. For one thing, the Hakim is a self-employed entrepreneur who makes unsubstantiated claims for his remedies and charges quite large sums of money for them. As such, he appears to orthodox eyes to be little better than a huckster or confidence trickster. (The critic may object that some allopathic remedies are of dubious value, and this is true, but there exists a complex and sophisticated system of legal controls encompassing product licences, clinical trials, and the Committee on Safety of Medicines, whose task is to ensure that false claims are not made and preparations are, at the least, not harmful.)

All Hakims practising in Britain, however well-intentioned or skilful, are undoubtedly breaking several laws. A doctor might turn a blind eye to this, but he would be foolhardy to identify himself personally with the activity. British doctors are expressly forbidden to collaborate with an unregistered practitioner in any way which could be construed as a partnership, and any doctor who did so would run the risk of being struck off the register.

At present, therefore, we can only say that collaboration would be valuable theoretically, but the practical problems of bringing it about are difficult to overcome. In the meantime, it is important that the orthodox practitioner should realize that his patient is not 'his' patient alone, but is probably receiving concurrent treatment from other sources, whether he admits it or not.

In the case of religious healers who do not prescribe drugs, the objections to collaboration are not so great, since the law is not being broken. (Anyone can set up as a healer: what is illegal is any claim to be a doctor of medicine, and especially the prescribing of remedies within the scope of the Medicines Act.) There is nothing to prevent a psychiatrist collaborating with a spiritual healer, hypnotherapist, or exorcist if he thinks fit, nor with a Molvi or Mullah or Guru. Such collaboration is of benefit not only to the patient, but also in broadening the outlook of the doctor. The obstacles are psychological, and they are greatest when the doctor perceives a conflict between 'pure science' and 'pure magic' — as he might in the case of the Devi or Obeah Man. This is exemplified in the following story from a West Indian island.

A health visitor was worried about a baby that was failing to thrive, the reason being that its mother refused to wean it on to solid food. Despite repeated explanations, she persisted in keeping the baby on the bottle, and told the Health Visitor that its weakness was due to an evil spirit. She knew this because the Obeah Woman had told her so. Eventually it seemed that the baby would die, so the health visitor in desperation plucked up her courage and went to talk to the Obeah Woman herself. The latter was not at all defensive, and in fact seemed pleased to be approached by a fellow-professional, and at the end of a long conversation the health visitor was able to state her own point of view about this particular case. The next time the baby was brought to the clinic it was obviously thriving.

'Not on the bottle any more?'

'No, Obeah Woman say bottle is bad.'

'But what about the evil spirit?'

'Obeah Woman very clever, discovered evil spirit getting into baby from bottle!'

Was this an example of successful collaboration? The health visitor thought so, and so did most of her colleagues at the seminar in which this story was told. A consultant psychiatrist who was present took a more jaundiced view. He protested that he spent a large amount of his professional time trying to stamp out superstition and educate people away from their beliefs in Obeah. In this case (he felt), by treating the Obeah Woman as a professional colleague her activities had been legitimized. Belief in evil spirits was reactionary and destructive in his experience, and all official health workers should set their faces firmly against it. By accepting her collaboration and allowing her to claim credit for the cure, the reputation of the Obeah Woman was enhanced, and her subsequent activities would be more difficult to control.

Both points of view have some validity, but the impartial observer may feel that the medical profession, more than most, should hesitate before using the word 'reactionary'.

It seems that doctors will be reluctant to work with either Hakims, whose role is similar to their own ('pretending to be proper doctors!'), or with those whose theoretical base is completely alien to them ('superstitious rubbish'). Between those two extremes, perhaps there is room for some links to be forged; or perhaps the reconciliation of orthodoxy with unorthodoxy must be initiated by someone else. Would clinical psychologists or social workers be able to approach this task with less restricted vision?

NOTE

1 Aslam's principal research was carried out in 1976–79 under the supervision of Professor S. S. Davis, Lord Trent Professor of Pharmacy at the University of Nottingham, supported by a research grant from the DHSS. Much of the fieldwork was undertaken in Bradford at the Transcultural Psychiatry Unit in collaboration with the present author among others. Detailed results are given in Aslam (1979) 'The Practice of Asian Medicine in the United Kingdom' PhD Thesis, University of Nottingham (unpublished) and Aslam and Davis (1979a, unpublished). Some of the major findings have been published in a series of papers (Aslam and Davis 1979b; Davis and Aslam 1979; Aslam *et al.* (in press). The present author is deeply indebted to Dr Aslam for permission to use his research as the basis for this chapter and to quote extensively from his work including portions not previously published. Dr Aslam is presently Lecturer in Clinical Pharmacy, University of Nottingham.

The 'Scientific' Practitioner's Response to 'Unscientific' Beliefs

We have seen that magical, religious, or superstitious beliefs are often expressed by mentally ill patients, and they are not necessarily evidence of psychosis (see Chapters 4, 12 and 14 above). How should the British practitioner respond to the patient who attributes his symptoms to witchcraft or supernatural intervention? The suggestion may be made by the patient, or by a relative. It may be mentioned openly, or (in the case of an educated person who has lived in Britain for many years) produced hesitantly or obliquely.

An intelligent Indian woman who had been brought up in Delhi in considerable affluence, now living a middle-class life in Britain, received treatment for depression for several months. In the psychiatrist's opinion her depression was mainly due to family relationships, and these were discussed in many joint sessions with her and her husband. Both were co-operative and seemed to be gaining insight. It was not until the tenth or eleventh session that she mentioned a cousin, still in India, who (she said) had always hated her and wished her harm. Very sheepishly she asked: Was it possible that her symptoms were caused by this enemy? Her husband looked very embarassed, and apologized to the doctor and changed the subject.

A fifty-three-year-old woman who had come to Britain from Jamaica at the age of twenty-five, consulted a psychiatrist because of intrusive 'bad words' that came into her head persistently. She received treatment for obsessive/compulsive disorder and depression. At the same time she applied to the Housing Department for a transfer to a different council estate, saying that she felt lonely because she had no Jamaican neighbours. She asked her psychiatrist for support in obtaining housing transfer priority on the grounds of her illness. Only after several months did she confide her belief that the house was haunted and that the intrusive thoughts were implanted by hostile spirits. In the meantime she had arranged several exorcism ceremonies at the house.

When something like this is revealed after months of treatment, the practitioner may feel that he has misjudged the situation from the start (which is always irritating), and that he should revise his diagnosis. Not necessarily so: his diagnosis may be quite correct, though it is true that he has been missing an important insight. How should he react? There is no universally 'right' response, but there are some wrong ones. Should he ignore it? No — because it is, after all, part of the clinical picture, and if the question were not important to the patient it would not have been raised. Should he dismiss it as nonsense, or laugh? Not unless he judges that this would be the most reassuring thing he could do. Should he take it seriously and pretend that he shares the belief in witchcraft or ghosts (assuming that he does not), and try to devise a magical protection against the magical threat? This is tempting. He could say, for example, that spells cast by a relative abroad could not possibly be effective since 'it is well known that spells do not work across water' — and if this statement were made with enough confidence it would probably be accepted. Or he could provide the patient with some kind of talisman, a material object, impregnated with the power of his own authority and charisma, which if placed on the mantlepiece at home would guard the patient against the evil influence. (Absurd as it may seem, that is exactly what doctors do very often provide — the magical object being, of course, a bottle of pills.) Taken to extremes, this line of approach conjures up images of the psychiatrist wearing a sorcerer's cloak, muttering incantations over a steaming cauldron, summoning demons to drive out demons, indulging a taste for amateur theatricals — and no doubt justifying it to his colleagues with phrases about meeting the patient 'where he is' and conducting therapy 'at the appropriate level'.

There are two objections to this. First, it is dishonest. That might not trouble the doctor too much, since in other circumstances he probably prescribes placebos with a clear conscience. More important, it is not what the patient wants from him. If the patient believed that magic of that kind would solve the problem, he would not have gone to the doctor but to some other kind of healer. Indeed, it is very likely that he has already consulted a magical or religious healer or is doing so concurrently with his medical treatment, and they are better equipped to carry out magical procedures impressively than any practitioner of Western medicine. The patient has come to the Western scientific doctor because he wants Western scientific medicine, and even if he does not have very much faith in it he is prepared to give it a try. For the scientific doctor to act so far outside his allotted role would be confusing, alarming, or ridiculous. If there is a 'right' response, it must be in terms of a compromise. The practitioner may be able to 'translate' the patient's concepts into his own conceptual framework. Suppose, for example, a patient says he is haunted by his grandfather's ghost. When the full story emerges, it transpires that his grandfather died some months ago, the patient knew that he was ill and intended to visit him, but kept putting it off, and did not learn about the death in time even to attend the funeral. He failed in his obligations during life, and his absence from the funeral was an unforgivable omission. Already we can see that 'haunted by grandfather's ghost' is a description we can accept figuratively, if not literally: we are in agreement about the cause of the symptoms, though one party may visualize a disembodied spirit floating in the air while the other would locate it in the mind.[1]

Or suppose that a young bride living with her in-laws says she is being poisoned by the witchcraft of a jealous sister-in-law. We may find that the sister-in-law is indeed jealous and spiteful, and is poisoning the atmosphere in the house in subtle ways that the poor bride cannot identify specifically but senses intuitively.

Not all ideas can be translated so easily. The notion that pain can be caused by an evil-minded person sticking pins into a wax effigy, at a distance and unknown to the victim, seems wholly incredible and indeed it is probably nonsense. Yet we are not forced to dismiss it out of hand. Telepathy is a phenomenon for which there is quite a lot of evidence. If it is possible to 'transmit' a thought or image and have it picked up by another person's mind, might it be possible to transmit a sensation of discomfort, or anxiety, or pain? Many orthodox Chrisitans believe that by praying for someone who is ill, they may influence the outcome of the illness: so why not the opposite too? There is no need for the practitioner to believe this wholeheartedly: in order to find common ground to keep a dialogue going, it is only necessary to refrain from ridicule or too-rigid disbelief.

In all these examples, the main differences between the magical and the psychological explanation is in terms of what is happening in the patient's head. The magical explanation can be represented as:

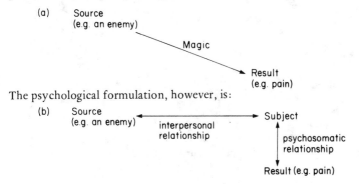

(a)   Source
        (e.g. an enemy)

                        Magic

                                    Result
                                    (e.g. pain)

The psychological formulation, however, is:

(b)   Source   Subject
        (e.g. an enemy) interpersonal
                         relationship   psychosomatic
                                        relationship

                                    Result (e.g. pain)

The difference is important, because in the first diagram the only ways to block the effect (i.e. relieve the pain), are to neutralize the source or to counteract the magical process; but in the second diagram there are other places in the sequence at which it is possible to make a therapeutic intervention. The second diagram could be expanded to any required degree of complexity, e.g.:

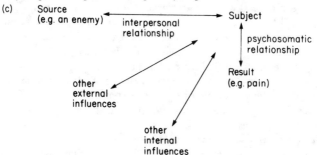

Once we start to visualise this kind of equilibrium, we can see a whole range of therapeutic possibilities.

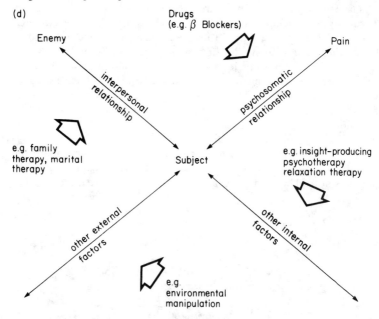

We have to try to translate the patient's concepts (a) into our own (d). Having made this translation for our own benefit, is it always necessary to present that translation to the patient, and insist on using it in all subsequent discussion? Not necessarily. This may be the point at which we meet conceptual and linguistic obstacles, since the habit of intro-spection is a cultural variable (Chapter 10). In less individualistic cultures people are less inclined to contemplate what is happening inside their own heads. So it may not be helpful to say to the man who is haunted by his grandfather's ghost 'There is no ghost — it is in your mind — you have a guilty conscience'. Instead, we might ask him what he thinks he ought to do to make his grandfather happy and allow his spirit to rest in peace. If he says that he should make a pilgrimage to the grave and carry out some propitiatory ritual, or erect a monument, or make provision for the widow, we would then check these proposals against our own translated version of the problem, and if they seemed to make good sense we could advise him to go ahead. In this way we would have succeeded in working within his terms of reference without stepping out of our own.

NOTE

1   I am indebted to Dr Roger Ballard for this example which, although fictitious in detail, is characteristic.

Practical Problems in Providing a Mental Health Service for Ethnic Minorities[1]

LANGUAGE

A reliable psychiatric diagnosis cannot be made unless the patient is interviewed in his own language by someone who knows what to look for. Even patients who speak enough English to communicate in every-day situations are likely to lose fluency in the stress of a medical or psychiatric interview. They may appear confused or deluded. Incoherence, hesitancy, and poverty of expression cannot readily be distinguished from psychotic thought disorder, depressive retardation, or cognitive impairment, so in 'making allowances' for linguistic defects the practitioner can easily miss important diagnostic pointers.

The problem is most obvious in relation to immigrants from Asia, and it has been avoided in recent years in most British mental hospitals by utilizing the services of junior doctors who came to Britain from India or Pakistan for postgraduate training. Their help has been invaluable. Nonetheless their presence, even if it continues in the future, does not solve all problems. It would be an unusual Asian doctor who was equally fluent in Hindi, Urdu, Punjabi, Pushtu, Bengali, and Gujarati (to name only the six commonest languages), let along their regional dialect variations. Linguistic variety within the Indian subcontinent is as great as it is in Europe, and to ask a doctor from Bombay to under-stand a peasant from Mirpur is like expecting an Edinburgh professor to understand a Spanish fisherman. In some ways the difference is greater, because throughout the Indian subcontinent the differences in *social class* between doctor and peasant are much wider than they are in Europe — they lead totally different lives and have different attitudes, beliefs, and values. Britain is far from egalitarian, but the middle-class doctor and the working-class patient have more shared experiences, and more chance of communicating with each other, than would be the case in India. Moreover, the Asian trainee psychiatrist in the British mental hospital may be occupying a fairly junior position, and to place complete diagnostic responsibility on a doctor whose psychiatric experience is a matter of months is not fair to either patient or doctor.

What about the more senior Asian doctor, who has been in Britain longer and holds a post as consultant or general practitioner? (There are also now a few social workers, probation officers, psychologists and nurses in equivalent positions.) Cannot they now assume responsibility? The answer is that they have an enormous potential contribution, but there are still some problems, including linguistic diversity and social class barriers and the possibility of 'overadaptation' which will be discussed later (Chapter 26). But how many of these people really wish to focus their professional attention on immigrant problems? The immigrant who is a member of a profession often prefers to present himself as a professional rather than an immigrant. Bearing in mind the insults to which every coloured person in Britain is exposed, and the struggle which the intelligent and educated black or brown man has in establishing himself in middle-class white society, it is understandable if he does not always choose to identify with the 'peasant' in the 'ghetto', with whom he has little in common except skin colour. The task of providing a service cannot be left entirely to him.

In Bradford we have been fortunate in being able to put together a clinical team which is not only multidisciplinary but multilingual, and for most of the languages required routinely there is a member of the team who can speak directly to the patient. He or she communicates *on behalf of the team*, which is not the same thing as *interpreting for the team*: the critical difference being that the person asking the questions understands their significance and the importance of the answers, and participates in diagnostic decision-making. The composition and work of this team is described in Appendix 4.

INTERPRETERS

It is unlikely that such a team could be brought into existence in every place where one would be useful, and it is inconceivable that any team could cover every language it might meet. Regretfully, we are obliged to consider the use of interpreters, even though this reduces diagnostic precision very greatly, sometimes to the level of guesswork. The interpreter may be a member of the patient's own family or circle, or an outsider brought in for the purpose by the practitioner. Both have drawbacks. It is the author's own view that *under no circumstances should children be asked to interpret medical details for their parents.* This practice is widespread and some writers have recommended it (e.g. Richie 1964) but it appears to us to be unethical, unprofessional, uncivilised and totally unacceptable. An adult relative or friend is less objectionable, but if he has no familiarity with medical and psychiatric matters he will find his task very difficult, and may intrude consciously or unconsciously his own interpretation of the problem, or report not what the patient says, but what he thinks he means (Henley 1979). Distortion may even be deliberate, as in the reported case in which the interview was tape-recorded and translated impartially later, when it was found that the interpreter had said: 'The doctor is asking you if you hear voices. Now, if you say that you are, he will take you to hospital and lock you up'. The interpreter must accept a code of confidentiality no less strict than that of the doctor, and it may be necessary to explain this and give specific assurances. In medicolegal matters, the friendly interpreter who comes with the patient is not acceptable, and an impartial one must be found, possibly from a distance. Confidentiality and impartiality are problems with the rarer languages. If there is only a small number of people in the neighbour-hood who speak, e.g. Ukrainian, Pushtu, or Vietnamese, it is wise to assume that they all know each other. Even if there are, say, a thousand Bengali-speakers in a city of half a million, it may be that those thousand form an enclosed community like a village within the city — and villages are notorious for gossip.

The appointment of official medical interpreters has not been given high priority in most Health Districts, even those with large non-English-speaking populations. Many hospitals have none at all, and rely on relatives, or personnel employed in the hospital in some other capacity who happen to have the required language. It is not surprising that when a survey of relevant Health Authorities was carried out in 1978, nearly all the respondents mentioned language as a major obstacle to health care (Wandsworth CRC 1978; Bhatti 1976). In some places where there are paid interpreters they are all part-timers, appointed by administrators in particular sectors, and paid on a lower clerical grade. There are no agreed selection criteria, no training, and very little monitoring of their activities. No policies have been formulated, and each department tends to work in isolation from the rest. In other places a person known to have the language is called in on request on a contract basis.

Most interpreters describe themselves as linguistic technicians. They are (they say) like human computers whose task is to give an accurate and undistorted rendering from one language to another in a wholly impersonal manner. Bearing in mind all the linguistic and conceptual pitfalls which have been mentioned in earlier chapters, we may doubt if this 'computer model' can ever be satisfactory in psychiatry. Even in other specialities the concept is probably naive. Probably the sort of thing that happens in practice is that the doctor says, 'Tell her that she has to come into hospital'. The answer comes back, 'She says that she does not want to come into hospital'. What happens next? Possibly the doctor says something like, 'Please try to find out why she says that, and see if you can persuade her'. The reasons why an Asian patient might be reluctant to enter hospital could be both personal and cultural. They are to do with the patient's perceptions of the hospital, and of themselves. The interpreter is being asked to explain to the patient how the doctor sees the situation, and explain to the doctor how the patient sees it. Already, even in this simple exchange, we are in the business of cultural interpretation, and have gone far beyond the linguistic computer concept. The patient is not talking to the doctor *through* the interpreter: he is talking *to* the interpreter (Price 1975). It is with the interpreter, not with the doctor, that the patient is developing personal rapport (or not, as the case may be). Similarly, the doctor is not always talking *to* the patient *through* the interpreter, but is quite often talking *to* the interpreter *about* the patient. Proponents of the 'linguistic computer' model will say this should not happen: if it does, we are placing on the interpreter a responsibility which he or she has not been selected or trained to accept. Yet it is difficult to see how it can be avoided, and if it is what does happen, interpreters should be selected and trained accordingly. What kind of training should such people receive? They must be fluently bilingual to start with but this is not a sufficient criterion, any more than ability to read English is an adequate qualification for a secretary. They should have the sort of educational background and personal characteristics that we would expect in any other important Health Service employee. Like medical secretaries, they should be given background knowledge of the meaning of medical terms, and the conventions and ethics of medical situations. They need to understand how patients feel, and have a working knowledge of the organization of that part of the service in which they are employed, so that they can answer patient's questions and reassure them. Their training must give them sufficient confidence to speak up boldly when they perceive that the two sides are misunderstanding each other. It is not always easy to tell a consultant that he is on the wrong track altogether because he has failed to see the significance of some point of cultural difference; nor is it easy for the consultant to accept such correction until he has learned to regard the interpreter as a professional colleague whose competence and acumen may be trusted. The interpreter should work with the same clinical team long enough for this to happen (Henley 1979; Bal 1981; Price 1975).

This kind of specialist service would be a far cry from the ad hoc arrangements currently in use, and would go some way towards making the mental health services accessible to non-English speaking patients. (It need not be applicable solely in psychiatry: the needs are almost as great in obstetric and paediatric departments, and in all types of social work, and there are similar problems in the legal sphere). The person described above is a specialist, as occupational therapists, physio-therapists, and radiographers are specialists: he or she would expect to be paid on a scale consistent with professional status and expertise. An interpreter service of this kind does not exist anywhere in Britain, though there have been some recent developments in the right direction in East London (Habershon, Tower Hamlets: personal communication). In Australia a service established in 1977 in New South Wales is re-portedly very successful and may expand elsewhere. In this project twenty-nine men and women who were bilingual and had previous experience in health or welfare work were given a course of training, and a year later they were seeing 600 patients per week.

> 'The interpreters not only help with direct communication between staff and patient but they also play an important role in relieving anxiety among patients and helping them with social problems. In some hospitals the interpreters scan the lists for migrant patients, for even those who can speak reasonable English find themselves very disorientated once in hospital.'   (Medical News 28.6.79)

In the present political and economic climate in Britain it is unlikely that DHSS will take any initiative to encourage such a development in Britain, and the onus is on local Health Authorities. It would not be expensive, would relieve a lot of distress among patients and frustration among staff, and would probably save money in the long run (see also Bal 1981).

Whatever arrangements may be made for interpreting, there is a great advantage in the practitioner himself taking the trouble to learn a little of the language commonly required. It is unlikely to be sufficient for reliable diagnosis, let alone therapy; but it helps if one can follow the gist of a conversation while it is taking place, without having to wait for the translation every time.

A few phrases, however badly pronounced, signal to the patient that the practitioner is at least making some effort in his direction; and if the practitioner makes himself look slightly ridiculous in the process, so much the better for both parties.

NAMES

In Britain, the rest of Europe, and the West Indies, names are standard-ized in form, comprising a surname (father's name if the parents are married, mother's if not) preceded by one or more forenames. This convention is not observed in all other parts of the world, and is not always clearly understood. Asian immigrants (including Vietnamese and Chinese) may give their names in a different order; it is not always customary for a wife to take her husband's name on marriage, or for children to have a name in common with their parents. Personal names, family names, caste names and appellations such as Singh or Kaur (which properly speaking are not names but titles) may be muddled, and this can produce untraceable records or two sets of records for the same patient. A list is given in Appendix 2, and useful guidance is contained in a recent handbook (Henley 1979). It is good practice to record some other identifying data such as father's full name, or birthplace, in order to avoid confusion between two or three patients who are all called (for example) Mohammed Khan. If in doubt how to address someone, it is sensible to ask. Dr David Smith probably does not relish being addressed as 'Smith', nor as 'Doctor David': patients do not like being addressed inappropriately either, though most will be too polite to object. Pronunciation is also important. Anyone who hears his own name repeatedly mispronounced feels irritation, and may interpret it as a sign of disinterest or contempt (perhaps with justification, though the intention may not be conscious). This applies just as much to names like Zubrycki or Wizniewski.

HOSPITAL ROUTINE

A patient admitted to a hospital ward in which he is unable to communicate with anyone at all is likely to feel apprehensive and tense. With the best of intentions one can hardly prevent such a patient being alarmed by unfamiliar and incomprehensible routines, or bored to distraction by social isolation. In such a situation, the strategy most people usually adopt is to observe what other people are doing, and copy them. In a psychiatric ward this can cause complications. Even a patient who genuinely wants to conform to the expectations of the institution can 'get into trouble' in innumerable ways due to misunderstandings about eating or toilet habits, religious observances, or behaviour towards other patients. Many misunderstandings can be avoided if nurses are aware of cultural norms and customs; the need for education of staff is slowly being recognised, and the handbook *Asian Patients in Hospital and at Home* (Henley 1979) is a useful introduction.

Lack of common language debars non-English speaking patients from most therapeutic activities in a psychiatric ward. They cannot talk through their problems with staff, nor participate in group activities. Occupational therapy is a meaningless concept to most Asians.

Hospitals (of all types) are particularly difficult for the young Indian or Pakistani girl who has not been in Britain long and has never before been separated from her extended family. Her emotional security and indeed her sense of personal identity are derived from her family membership. The family's dealings with authority have always been handled by her elders. She is not accustomed to *existing, as an individual person, on her own*. Whatever the nature of her illness, admission to hospital is likely to produce secondary complications.

Another vulnerable patient is the refugee for whom the walls of the institution and the loss of personal freedom evoke traumatic memories. Elderly people who are confused in their own homes usually become even more disorientated in a strange environment, and this effect is exacerbated if verbal communication is impossible.

FOOD

Hospital catering managers all probably know that Hindus do not eat beef, and Muslims and Jews do not eat pork; but in some cases that seems to be all they do know. In fact, some Hindus and Jains are totally vegetarian and a few are vegan. Sikhs, while not prohibited by religion from eating beef, often refuse it. Apart from Bengalis, few Indians eat fish regularly. It is perhaps not surprising that some hospitals take the easy way out and treat all Asians as vegetarians. Institutional catering is seldom excellent, but institutional *vegetarian* catering is usually totally unimaginative. The diet often consists of eggs and cheese in various combinations. Unfortunately cheese, while acceptable to all but vegans, is unfamiliar as a constituent of Asian cooking, and the taste is not always appreciated. For a strictly orthodox Muslim or Jew, it is not enough to avoid pork products: *all* meat may be unacceptable unless the animal has been killed under Hal'al or Kosher conditions, and in theory all food should be prepared in utensils kept specially for the purpose and never used for prohibited materials. The majority of Muslims and Jews in Britain will accept some compromises on these restrictions, but a few will not. Most are suspicious of made-up dishes in which they cannot identify the constituents.

There are no easy solutions to these problems. It is probably unrealistic to expect a hospital, or group of hospitals, to provide a special kitchen (though this was provided in the past in Leeds, for Jews). If a plated meals service operates in the hospital, it is possible for special meals to be obtained from an outside contractor, either locally or wholesale, for re-heating on the premises: another alternative is to make it clear to patient's relatives that they are at liberty to bring prepared meals in daily, and use the ward kitchen to re-heat them. None of these arrangements are very satisfactory, and in hospitals where dietary problems are encountered frequently, pressure should be brought to bear on the Catering Officer to seek better alternatives.

ENTITLEMENT TO NHS TREATMENT

Under legislation due for implementation in October 1982, restrictions will be placed on the use of the NHS by visitors to Britain. Hitherto, ever since the inception of the service in 1948, the so-called 'Good Samaritan' policy has operated, whereby emergency treatment was provided without charge. 'Emergency Treatment' was never closely defined, but was usually interpreted as applying to conditions that were not present or apparent before arrival. This was irrespective of any reciprocal arrangements that exist with some other countries.

The new proposals are ostensibly directed against abuse of the system by visitors who come specifically to obtain free treatment for preexisting illness. (The cost of a transatlantic air fare is small by comparison with medical charges in America.) The government estimates a saving of some $6 million per year (Fowler 1982) but most critics consider that the cost of operating a screening procedure will exceed the savings. It is proposed that all persons registering for hospital treatment be asked three questions to determine their entitlement, followed up by further enquiries in doubtful cases. Exemption from charges will be granted to anyone who has been in Britain for more than one year, and to various other categories which are listed in Appendix 6.

Apart from its dubious cost-effectiveness, the new legislation looks at first sight to be a reasonable measure. In fact it is objectionable on several grounds. It will cause particular hardship to overseas students who become ill in their first year, and to families who invite a relative to visit them in Britain if that relative becomes ill here. More important, the questions which receptionists are to ask will cause offence to many, and will be interpreted by members of ethnic minorities in particular as evidence of discrimination. There were examples of this under the former system: in 1980 a hospital administrator in London was quoted as saying:

> 'It's just a matter of common sense, whether we go on their being foreign, or their colour, or whatever . . . we deal with it here on an ad hoc basis. A lot of these people will obviously say they've been here for years, but only their passports can clarify the matter.'
> (JCWI Briefing, December 1981)

The practice of asking all Asian patients attending hospital to produce their passports was standard in Leicester in the past, until ruled unlawful under the Race Relations Act. Such practices may become common and legally defensible under the new regulations, and if so patients who are legally entitled to use the service will be inhibited from doing so. A particular problem arises for psychiatric patients who are to be treated free if compulsorily detained but not if admitted informally: the consequences of this should be carefully monitored.

NOTE

1   See also Rack 1977, 1978.

Racial Differences in Response to Drugs[1]

There is at least a possibility that members of different races[2] may have different reactions to some of the drugs that are used in psychiatric treatment. The issue is of some importance because if the margin of safety of a drug is small, variation due to racial differences may be dangerous. Even if not dangerous, unpleasant side-effects may be produced if subjects are given more of a drug than they require, affecting compliance (and therefore effectiveness) (Binder and Levy 1981).

Most of the evidence comes from comparisons of average doses used to treat patients in different parts of the world. For example, American psychiatrists tend to use higher doses of phenothiazines to treat schizophrenics than European clinicians, who in turn use higher doses than those working in Third World countries. The same trend appears with antidepressants and anxiolytic drugs, but, being anecdotal, the evidence allows no control over variables such as diagnosis, measurements of change, and availability or expense of medication.

A few studies have been reported in which control over these factors was attempted. One of the first was carried out by Denber and his colleagues (Denber and Bente 1967). They compared the doses of butyrylperazine needed to achieve a therapeutic effect in American (Manhattan) and West German (Erlangen) patients suffering from schizophrenia. The mean daily dose needed by the Manhattan patients was 126 mg compared with only 26 mg in the Erlangen group. The therapeutic response was mediocre in Manhattan and excellent in Erlangen, while side effects were more troublesome in Erlangen (despite the lower dosage). Later, using more stringent controls the same authors found the mean daily dose required to treat Manhattan schizophrenics to be 90 mg compared with 40 mg in a matched population at Erlangen (Denber et al. 1962). In a later study of Haloperidol the average daily dose used in Manhattan was 14.6 mg compared with 8.8 mg for a group of Belgian patients (Denber and Collard 1962). Itil examined therapeutic, toxic and electro-encephalographic (EEG) response to various neuro-leptic drugs in Turkish and American patients. Much greater improve-ment took place in the Turkish patients, who also had a higher incidence of side effects. Computer analysis of EEG also showed different effects in the two groups. Itil has also studied the effect of Diazepam on the EEGs of healthy Turkish and American volunteers. He found the same qualitative changes in EEG recordings but the Turkish sample exhibited greater change per dose of drug than the American subjects (Itil 1975).

The problem with inter-country comparisons is that there may be differences in the clinical settings (standards of hospital care, staff/patient ratio, concurrent psychotherapy and activation, etc). A study which avoids that has been reported by Raskin and Crook (1975). They examined the effects of Imipramine and Chlorpromazine in 714 depressed in-patients at five American psychiatric hospitals and found that black patients improved more and seemed to do better than white patients on the same dose of anti-depressants. Among whites there was no significant difference between men and women, but black men seemed more responsive to Imipramine while black women seemed more responsive to Chlorpromazine.

This sort of comparison is still open to scepticism because the estimations of improvement may be biased by cultural factors. There is, however, some evidence that a drug may be differently handled — i.e. its rate of absorption, or detoxification, or excretion, may be different, and these differences in pharmacokinetics would affect the plasma concentration and the concentration available at the site of action. A few studies of plasma concentration have been reported. Zeigler and Biggs (1977) reported the effects of several variables including race on plasma concentrations of two anti-depressants Amitriptyline and Nortriptyline in a group of black and white depressed patients; black patients had significantly higher levels of Nortriptyline than white patients. A study carried out in Bradford (see Note (1)) suggests that a similar difference may exist with another anti-depressant of the same group, Clomipramine. Figure 22 (1) shows some results representing the plasma levels over time after single 25 mg and 50 mg doses of Clomipramine in thirty British and fifteen Asian volunteers. Asians achieve higher peak levels after each dose and the peak difference at four hours (25 mg) and at two, four, eight, and twenty-four hours (50 mg) are significant. Calculation of the area under the curve (AUC) for each subject gives an indication of the total amount of drug present in the plasma over a twenty-four hour period and there is a significant difference in AUC between the groups after a 50 mg dose. A similar difference may be found with some phenothiazine drugs (Lewis *et al.* in press).

Figure 22 (1)

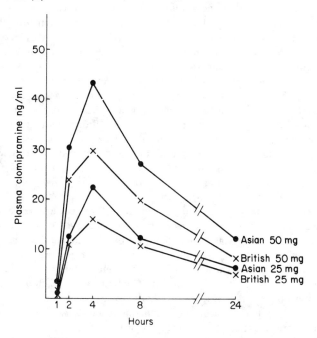

Mean plasma clomipramine concentration in 30 British
and 15 Asian subjects after single doses of 25 and 50 mg

The difference may be due to differences in absorption rates, but there may also be differences in the rate of breakdown or deactivation of a drug, or its excretion. An example of differential deactivation is provided by another antidepressant, Phenelzine. There are two alternative mechanisms whereby this drug is de-activated in the body, processes of either fast acetylation or slow acetylation. Everyone is either a fast or a slow acetyaltor; which one is a matter of genetics. Fast and slow acetylators occur in every group that has been studied but like blood groups they differ in incidence. Canadian Eskimos are 5 per cent slow and 95 per cent fast, whereas in Egypt the proportions are reversed (Whitford 1978). Since it is believed that the rate of acetylation affects drug efficacy it may be that a drug that is effective in one country is ineffective in another. Very little research has been done on this; a recent pilot survey showed that Indians/Pakistanis seem to be genetically similar to Europeans in this respect (Stevenson, Lewis, and Rack 1982 – unpublished).

If there are metabolic differences between races this need not surprise us, since other metabolic differences are already well known (most obviously the production of melanin pigment in the skin). We cannot be sure, however, that all metabolic differences between 'races' are purely genetic in origin. Differences in diet would affect absorption rates, and climatic differences may also be important. So also may previous exposure: Europeans and Americans are exposed to a wide variety of chemicals from an early age, including food additives, houeshold drugs (aspirin) and social drugs (nicotine and caffeine). The body responds to the presence of such compounds by developing detoxifying enzymes, which are not all specific to the particular compound. Some interesting evidence about this is provided by recent work on plasma concentrations of antipyrine (a compound which is easily measured) among a London population which included Asians and Gambians (Fraser *et al.* 1976). In the Londoners antipyrine half-life was shortened in smokers and lengthened in women taking oral contraceptives, and also in vegetarians (which included most of the Asians). In the Gambians it was prolonged by cola-nut chewing. In another antipyrine study (Branch *et al.* 1980) a group of Sudanese who had lived for at least two years in London were compared with other English subjects and with Sudanese in Sudan. The Sudanese in London reacted like other Londoners, not like other Sudanese.

Obviously a good deal of work remains to be done in this area. At present there is sufficient evidence to suggest that:

(1) When new drugs are introduced their efficacy and toxicity should be assessed in each separate ethnic or racial group. It is not sufficient to carry out controlled clinical trials in one country and then utilize the drugs world-wide without local confirmatory trials.

(2) The practitioner prescribing for members of other races should be prepared to use low doses and increase gradually if necessary. This recommendation certainly applies to tricyclic antidepressants in Asian subjects and it may well apply to other categories of drugs or other groups.

NOTES

1 For fuller details see Allen, Rack, and Vadaddi (1977), Lewis, Vadaddi, Rack, and Allen (1980), and Rack (1980). The author gratefully acknowledges the contributions of these co-authors on whose work the present chapter is largely based.

2 The term 'race' is used with the reservations mentioned in Chapter 2.

Repatriation

A person who is unhappy in Britain, or seems unable to cope, may decide that it would be a good idea to return to his or her country of origin, or someone else may suggest that they should do so.

There is a great deal of coming and going between Britain and the main emigrant countries. The idea of migration as a one-way, once-for-all process is quite outdated — certainly as far as India, Pakistan, and Bangla Desh are concerned. Very few Indians or Pakistanis remain in Britain for more than ten years without making at least one visit 'home' (Anwar 1979). The periods of absence range from a few months to several years, with a limiting factor that anyone who is away for more than two years runs a risk of being regarded as a new immigrant on re-entry.[1] Even children born in Britain are quite likely to spend some part of their childhood in the parental country of origin.[2]

Adults may choose to go 'home' for many reasons, including homesickness and illness. Frequently they do not decide beforehand exactly how long they will be away. For people who have retained their emotional ties with the extended family, the prospect of going back for good remains a perpetual possibility. Many elderly West Indian immigrants find that England seems to get less attractive, and decide to return.

In the context of all this coming and going it may be assumed that the vast majority of people who decide that they are not happy in Britain and wish to return to their country of birth, make their own arrangements to do so without seeking advice or assistance from anyone other than family and friends, and there are no statistics about the size of this group or their reasons for going.

Practitioners are likely to become involved when advice, financial assistance, or other action is required, in the following situations:

(1) The subject is unsure whether or not going home would be helpful, or has not considered the possibility, but is open to suggestions, advice, or persuasion.

(2) The subject thinks that his problems will be solved by going home, but is making this decision in a state of depression, anxiety, or distorted judgment through illness or other cause, and will probably regret it later if he goes.

(3) The suggestion comes not from the subject himself but from others who are apparently concerned for his happiness but may be mistaken or have ulterior motives.

(4) Financial assistance is required from public funds, and a case has to be made to obtain it.

(5) The rare case of the psychiatric patient who does not wish to go but should be compelled or persuaded to do so in his own interest. This can be done under Section 90 of the Mental Health Act, but is much more often achieved by persuasion.

It is the last of these categories, in which there is an element of compulsion or persuasive pressure, which demands the closest scrutiny. Perhaps the term 'repatriation' should be used only in this context, all other forms of assisted travel being given some less provocative label. In practice, however, the distinction may not be quite so clear-cut, since people who are confused or distressed can be talked into giving their assent to the recommendations of professional advisors (especially doctors). In such cases the pretence that the patient exercized his or her own unfettered judgement is a legal fiction: 'one may be allowed to speculate that consultants might see "voluntary" return as a way of getting rid of longstay patients of overseas origin, and it is therefore essential to make sure that patients are not pressurized into saying they want to go back'.[3] With this caveat in mind, the case for compulsory repatriation will be considered first, although as we shall see the numbers involved are very small.

COMPULSORY REPATRIATION OF PSYCHIATRIC PATIENTS

Statutory powers are vested in the Home Secretary under Section 90 of the Mental Health Act (1959). The relevant Section (as amended by Section 30 of Immigration Act 1971) states:

'90. If it appears to the Secretary of State*, in the case of any patient who is not patrial within the meaning of the Immigration Act 1971 who is receiving treatment for mental illness as an inpatient − (a) in a hospital in England and Wales: or (b) in a mental hospital within the meaning of the Mental Health (Northern Ireland) Act 1948, that proper arrangements have been made for the removal of the patient to a country or territory outside the United Kingdom,

* Secretary of State refers throughout to the Home Secretary

the Isle of Man and the Channel Islands for his care or treatment there and that it is in the interests of the patient to remove him, the Secretary of State may by warrant authorise the removal of the patient from the place where he is receiving treatment as aforesaid, and may give such directions as the Secretary of State thinks fit for the conveyance of the patient to his destination in that country or territory and for his detention in any place or on board any ship or aircraft until his arrival at any specified port or place in any such country or territory.'

The numbers of people repatriated in recent years under this act are given in *Table 23 (1)*

Table 23 (1) *Psychiatric patients transferred overseas under Section 90 of Mental Health Act 1959*

Total numbers		Countries to which transferred			
1970	8	Austria	1	Ireland	2
		Barbados	1	Israel	2
1971	6	Belgium	1	Italy	7
		Canada	1	New Zealand	1
1972	5	Colombia	1	Nigeria	6
		Czechoslovakia	1	Pakistan	2
1973	11	Dominica	1	Phillipines	1
		Finland	1	Poland	4
1974	11	France	2	Portugal	1
		Germany (FDR)	2	St. Kitts	1
1975	9	Grenada	1	Spain	1
		Guyana	1	Trinidad	1
1976	7 (to 31st Oct)	Hong Kong	3	United States	7
		Hungary	1	Yemen	1
Total	57	Indonesia	1	Yugoslavia	2
X̄	7.3				

(Adapted from *Hansard* 10.11.76.)

In November 1976 the then Minister of State at the Home Office (Lord Harris of Greenwich) stated:

'No action is in practice taken to remove a patient unless my right honourable friend* is first approached by the doctor responsible for the patient's treatment. Where admission is to be to a hospital over-seas for continued treatment my right honourable friend requires to

* The Home Secretary

see copies of the correspondence which the doctor has had with the authorities of the hospital to which it is proposed to admit him. Where, in the opinion of the doctor responsible, the patient is well enough to be discharged to the care of relatives abroad or treated as an out-patient, evidence is required that proper arrangements have been made and that the patient will be met by relatives or a doctor as appropriate, on his arrival in his own country. It is not unusual to find that a patient who requires in-patient treatment in this country can safely be treated in the community in his country of origin.'

(Hansard 10.11.76)

Despite these reassurances, some might feel that this legislation is open to abuse and could conceivably be used to dispose of a troublemaker. The author is not aware of any evidence of such abuse. Nonetheless it may be asked whether the legislation is just, or is necessary. Any forcible intervention in the life of an individual must be subjected to rigorous scrutiny, however loudly the interveners protest their good intentions, and sending someone away from the country is a very great intervention indeed.

In this chapter we are considering only situations in which repatriation is thought to be in the interest of the individual concerned. We are not concerned with repatriation as social policy, as advocated by certain political groups, nor with the deportation of people who have committed criminal offences. We may have views on these matters, and make them known through appropriate channels, but any professional involvement in criminal deportation cases (of which illegal entry and overstaying are the most common) is likely to be when an opinion is requested on behalf of someone threatened with deportation when there may be medical or social reasons to object to it. This is a different issue. Currently we are considering repatriation on the sole grounds that this is conceived to be in the best interest of the patient or client. The suspicion expressed by Lord Avebury (quoted above) is pertinent: ulterior motives such as: 'then at least he won't be bothering *us* any more' are insidious and understandable, but ethically inadmissable for anyone in a care-giving or advice-giving relationship.

In the author's opinion, as long as the law is applied in the manner described, and not very often, and in accordance with professional principles, and is kept under scrutiny, Section 90 repatriations can be justified. One can easily imagine a situation in which a person who has received psychiatric treatment in his own country, suffers a relapse while in Britain, and requires further treatment. He may be here as a student or short-term visitor. There could be several reasons — including language problems, and the absence of family — why treatment could not be given satisfactorily in Britain, and after consulting his doctor and his family it would seem right to send him home. But a patient suffering from confusion, or delusions of a psychotic nature, might not accept the need for transfer, and it is in such cases that reserve powers of compulsion are needed.

Some aspects of this legislation are unsatisfactory. Currently, it can be applied to an in-patient in a psychiatric hospital even if he is not detained there under any other section of the Mental Health Act. The vast majority of psychiatric patients are admitted to hospital informally, and are free to discharge themselves at any time. As it now stands, an application under Section 90 could be made in respect of an informal patient who could nullify it when the time came by discharging himself. Also it is not clear how much information is required from the other country or how it is obtained. The absence of any system of appeal is noteworthy.

These points were considered by an Ad-Hoc Committee set up in 1977 on the initiative of the then Community Relations Commission. This committee recommended that the use of Section 90 should be limited to patients detained under Treatment Orders (Sections 26, 60, and 65 of the Mental Health Act). Compulsory detention under these Sections is subject to quite stringent criteria, and patients so detained have the right of appeal to a Mental Health Tribunal. A Tribunal should be convened in all cases where repatriation is considered under Section 90, whether or not this is requested by the patient, and it should be the duty of the tribunal to ensure that transfer is in the patient's interest and that adequate arrangements have been made in the receiving country.

The Mental Health (Amendment) Bill currently under consideration includes recommendations which, while they fall short of the above proposals may make it easier for clinicians to adopt this procedure voluntarily as a code of good practice.

Currently the correct procedure under Section 90 is as follows:

(1) Application to the Home Office is unnecessary if the patient (whether or not accompanied by an escort) is able and willing to travel without powers of detention, and suitable arrangements for the journey have been made.

(2) In all other cases, application should be made in writing by the hospital authorities to the Home Office Immigration Department, 50 Queen Anne's Gate, London SW1H 9AT, stating:

    (a) that the patient is receiving treatment for mental illness as an in-patient;

    (b) that it is in the patient's interest to transfer him abroad, and why;

    (c) the arrangements which have been or could be made for the patient's care or treatment abroad, with copies of correspondence;

    (d) what arrangements have been made regarding passports and visas;

    (e) proposed travel arrangements if made;

    (f) whether an escort is necessary and can be provided.

(3) Travel reservations should *not* be confirmed until authorization under Section 90 has been issued.

(Summarized from DHSS Memorandum of Guidance on the Provisions under the Mental Health Act 1959 (1960) paras 277–78; and DHSS Memorandum on Psychiatric Hospital Services (1961) paras 4–7.)

CHILDREN

The repatriation of children can be arranged under Section 24 of the Child Care Act 1980, which states:

(1) Local Authority may, with the consent of the Secretary of State, procure or assist in procuring an emigration of any child in their care.

(2) The Secretary of State shall not give his consent under this Section unless he is satisfied that emigration would benefit the child and that suitable arrangements have been or will be made for the child's reception and welfare in the country to which he is going, that the parents or guardian of the child have been consulted, or that it is not practicable to consult them, and that the child consents.

(3) Provided that where a child is too young to form or express a proper opinion on the matter, the Secretary of State may consent to his emigration notwithstanding that the child is unable to consent thereto.

Practitioners (social workers in particular) may become involved in cases in which there is disagreement between parents or guardians, and the child's removal from Britain does not necessarily seem to be in the child's own interests. In such cases it may be necessary to seek a Care Order pending legal proceedings.

VOLUNTARY REPATRIATION AND FINANCIAL ASSISTANCE

Apart from Section 90 of the Mental Health Act there are no powers of compulsory repatriation unless a criminal offence has been committed, and then only in certain cases. Every other form of repatriation is voluntary, so it is a matter of obtaining financial assistance for someone who wishes to leave but requires help in doing so.

The statutory sources of financial assistance are Area Health Authorities, Supplementary Benefits Commission, and International Social Services. There is considerable confusion regarding these various sources, each of which applies different criteria which are not always fully understood even by the officials who operate them. An applicant for assistance is certain to need expert help in preparing his application, and may request this help from a social worker, community relations officer, solicitor, doctor, or any other person. The procedure is likely to be lengthy and can be frustrating.

All three sources have the following criteria in common:

(1) The applicant must want to go.
(2) He must have no prospect of being able to find sufficient money himself.
(3) Enquiries will be made in the receiving country to ensure that he is accepted there.

These conditions should be told to the applicant at the outset. If he does not accept them (e.g. because he does not wish his relatives to know he is going home 'as a failure') he cannot be assisted statutorily. He should also be told that he may not be permitted to re-enter Britain. The Immigration Rules on the rights of returning residents include the phrase: 'except one who received assistance from public funds towards the cost of leaving this country'. In the most recent amendment of the Rules (February 1980) it appears that Commonwealth citizens settled in Britain before January 1973 can return within two years even though they may have been helped to leave with public funds; but Commonwealth citizens settled after that date, and aliens, lose their right of return if they have received such assistance.

In practice, people who have been repatriated with public funds do seem to be able to re-enter Britain, which suggests that the screening process is not very efficient. All the same, the applicant for funds should be given this warning about re-entry.

HEALTH AUTHORITY FUNDS

There is no statutory provision for meeting the cost of voluntary repatriation from DHSS funds, but in the case of a patient who is or has recently been in hospital, if funds cannot be obtained from other sources, the Health Authority may apply to the DHSS for permission to use hospital funds for this non-statutory purpose and this may include the cost of an escort if necessary. This provision is part of a reciprocal arrangement with commonwealth countries and it is therefore properly applicable to commonwealth citizens only. The numbers assisted through this scheme amount to about twelve per year. Most are long-term patients and usually, but not always, psychiatric patients. The DHSS requires assurances that in the opinion of a consultant repatriation is in the patient's interest, and that appropriate facilities are available in the home country. The hospital is responsible for making those enquiries, which may be channelled through the High Commission of the country or through ISS (see below).

SUPPLEMENTARY BENEFITS COMMISSION

Applicants must be in receipt of or eligible to receive supplementary benefits. The criteria, as stated by the SBC, are:

(1) The person concerned has virtually no prospects of settling down and making a success of life in this country, whether because of physical or mental handicap, or sickness or for other reasons (excluding a temporary high level of unemployment in the locality).
(2) He is unlikely to find work and save up the fare, and the money is not available from other sources.
(3) He genuinely wishes to return home, with his dependents if any, and it seems to be in his best interests to do so.
(4) Payment of the fare will lead to an ultimate saving in public funds.

All four criteria must be satisfied. Guidance issued to local offices sets out the detailed information required by the headquarters branch, which is then responsible for all subsequent action on the application.[4]

To ascertain that repatriation is in the applicant's interests, the SBC makes enquiries about home circumstances through the High Commissions of the countries concerned. This sometimes takes a long time.

In practice, SBC is one of the most used sources of assistance. In the ten years 1966–75 assistance was given to an average eighty-four families per year (average of 163 individuals per year for which separate figures are available). Separate statistics for psychiatric patients or ex-patients are not kept, but they are thought to be a minority. The Commission has been known to refuse an applicant on the grounds that he was not eligible for supplementary benefit, having never worked in Britain. In another case, (a non-commonwealth citizen), it was stated that 'He will be required to sign an undertaking to repay to the Government of the UK the total amount advanced . . . as such an undertaking is an integral part of the procedure where repatriation is at public expense'. Such statements are wrong and should be challenged.

INTERNATIONAL SOCIAL SERVICE OF GREAT BRITAIN

This organization, the existence of which is not well known to all practitioners, provides perhaps the most effective source of assistance. It administers funds supplied by the Home Office under Section 29 of the Immigration Act 1971. These funds are basically intended for people who:

(1) Have come to the UK from abroad and were permitted to reside here, but have found it difficult to settle and wish to re-settle in an overseas country (excluding a European country).
(2) Are non-patrial. (In case of doubt about this, ISS can advise.)
(3) Have insufficient income to pay their own fares. Certain income limits are laid down. If the applicant has property or savings he may be expected to make a contribution towards the cost of his travel.
(4) Have prospects of satisfactory resettlement overseas.
(5) Have no intention of returning to reside in Britain.

Applications are considered from anyone who fulfils these criteria. Each applicant is interviewed by a social worker to discuss his plans. ISS has to be satisfied that repatriation is in the applicant's best interest, and usually undertakes enquiries in the receiving country through its own network of professional contacts, but this network is inevitably incomplete, and enquiries may take some time. Help may be given towards the cost of travel of the applicant and members of his family or household. Travel arrangements are made by ISS. There is no provision for any resettlement grant.[5]

In the six years up to March 1979, an average of 167 persons per year were assisted under Section 29 of the Immigration Act. Quite a lot of them are known to have had some form of mental breakdown while in Britain, but separate figures for psychiatric patients are not kept.

ISS may also be willing to help (within the limits of the organization's small budget) to obtain information from the receiving country when repatriation is being considered by some other channel.

GOVERNMENT OF THE RECEIVING COUNTRY

It may be worth contacting the High Commission or local Consular Office of the country concerned, to see whether they can be of any assistance in a particular case, e.g. by providing information or obtaining money from relatives in the home country, or by providing direct financial assistance. There does not seem to be any universal policy about this but it is worth trying.

REPATRIATION AS THERAPY: FOLLOW-UP STUDIES

Apart from criminal deportation, repatriation cannot be assisted with funds from any of the above sources unless it can be shown that return is in the person's interest, and this is in any case an ethical requirement. We must therefore be as sure as possible that the move is actually helpful, and be prepared to advise against it if not. A patient may feel that his anxiety, depression, or feelings of persecution are due to malignant influences in Britain, whereas he would in fact lose them quite quickly if given appropriate treatment, and such treatment may be available here but not in his own country. The initiative for re-patriation may come from family or friends, and it can happen that a family finds itself embarrassed by the behaviour of a mentally ill member and wants him 'out of the way' (believing that his condition is in any case, hopeless). The patient or relatives may feel that the condition would respond to religious or magical treatments, or to a change of environment. In some cases they may be right, but not always. For example, a teenage girl who had diabetes and was also behaving in a way that her parents disapproved of, was sent back to India by them against the author's advice. The parents were convinced that a local healer could cure her diabetes, and that her rebellious behaviour (which they construed as madness) would be cured by an arranged marriage. She died in India a few months later. In another case, a husband took his depressed wife back to Pakistan where he divorced her on the grounds that she was mad (i.e. had received psychiatric treatment in Britain) and returned to Britain himself with a second wife. A difficult dilemma is provided by the overseas student who suffers an acute stress-related breakdown. Repatriation may relieve his symptoms instantly – indeed, in some cases he is quite well by the time he steps off the plane at the other end – but if this is achieved at the cost of his whole future career, it is a heavy price to pay.

In cases where there is no overt psychiatric problem and financial assistance with fares is sought on social grounds, the applicant will usually be regarded as the best judge of his own situation. Probably every Community Relations Officer has a file of letters of thanks from people who have been helped in this way when circumstances made life in Britain very difficult for them. Examples provided by Bradford CRC include a sixty-six-year-old Sikh who was on the point of returning to India and had his savings stolen; a thirty-year-old Bangla Deshi with intractable asthma attributed to the British climate; a Pakistani woman whose husband died suddenly leaving her with young children and no other relatives in Britain; and a Jamaican family in which the parents were worried about the moral welfare of their children. Reviewing the cases in the CRC files we have noticed however that in a significant number of them a member of the family was or had been under psychiatric treatment and this was used as evidence in support of their application. Whoever offers advice and assistance has a professional obligation to make his own judgement about the client's long-term interests.

Very few follow-up studies have been reported. In a paper entitled 'The consequences of unplanned repatriation', Burke (1973) reviewed a series of two hundred patients in the admission ward of Bellevue Mental Hospital, Jamaica, among whom he found sixteen (8 per cent) who had previously received treatment in British mental hospitals. He refers to these as 'repatriates', though it is not stated that they were ill when they went home, or were forced to return, but many of them said they had been advised or persuaded to go. The mean interval between returning to Jamaica and being admitted to Bellevue was 2.4 years. Burke claimed that sufferers from what he called the 'repatriate syndrome' were clinically distinguishable from other patients, being solitary, unresponsive, and depressed, 'more like the chronic mental hospital patients in England than like mentally ill patients in Jamaica'. Fourteen of the sixteen were suffering from schizophrenia, and in most cases the same diagnosis had been made in Britain (the case notes from Britain were obtained for comparison). The author surmises that repatriation may have been advised in the hope of avoiding further breakdowns, in which case for those patients the hope was not fulfilled. However, the methodology of this study excludes patients who did not break down again, for whom repatriation may have been beneficial. The conclusion that 'No support for optimism about repatriation as therapy was found' therefore appears somewhat disingenuous. However, Burke has additional figures, as yet unpublished, that lend greater support to this conclusion (Burke, personal communication).

Mahy (1976) reported a study in which he noted from 1968 onwards a 'rapid increase' in his psychiatric clinic in Barbados of patients who had been to Britain. He collected data on 100 men and 100 women who had gone to Britain without any previous history of mental illness, who had received in-patient psychiatric treatment in Britain, and had then returned and were accessible to his survey (in Barbados, Grenada, and adjacent islands). Presumably most of them were his patients but this is not stated. He excluded those who at the time of the survey were too deluded or thought-disordered to be questioned. One hundred and four (52 per cent) of the sample said they had been 'either repatriated or strongly advised to return' (but see *Table 23(1)* above). Many now regretted it, and 128 (64 per cent) wished they could return to Britain. Many had relatives there. As with the previous study, these findings cannot tell us anything about the successful ones who have avoided further contact with psychiatric services, but they do indicate a large number of repatriated patients who remain ill, or relapse, after returning home.

In Mahy's series, the first illness had occurred in Britain within two years of arrival in 45 per cent of cases, which accords with the findings of, for example, Gordon (1965) and Hemsi (1967). In those classified as severely ill, a significant finding was that 79 per cent had been living alone and 6 per cent said that they never visited English homes and 'felt like outsiders' — whereas in a control sample only 12 per cent lived alone and only 17 per cent were culturally isolated. Plainly, repatriation is no panacea even for those suffering social and cultural isolation which might reasonably have been regarded as a causative factor in their illness.

There are no comparable studies published from the Indian sub-continent. In most parts of India, Pakistan, and Bangla Desh the psychiatric services are such that epidemiological surveys are impossible. Possibly there are many for whom the support of the family more than outweighs the absence of medical treatment, who are better off at home than in Britain where they would be permanently or recurrently in hospitals; but we can be fairly sure that there are many others who are worse off. Certainly for those disorders (e.g. chronic schizophrenia) for which long-term maintenance medication is required to avoid relapses, a return to India, Pakistan, Bangla Desh, (and many other countries) should not be recommended unless they are fortunate enough to live in a city with adequate medical services and wealthy enough to afford them.

A further point is made by both Burke and Mahy, and applies also to Asians. The migrant who returns home because of illness is regarded as having failed. He has wasted his opportunities: the hopes of his family have not been fulfilled. He will not necessarily receive a warm welcome.

'Many of our psychotic patients might have requested repatriation during their paranoid delusions and are still regretting it because in many cases they were not welcomed home.'   (Mahy 1976)

'In fact the mental sequelae are accompanied by severe stigma in society and a worsening of the mental state. This is typified by depressive features, lack of motivation, difficulty in obtaining employment, and a chronic course [of illness].'   (Burke 1973)

The British doctor who advises his patient to go home may have a picture in his mind of a close-knit warm-hearted rural community, or a sun-drenched beach where fruit falls from the trees. If life in those

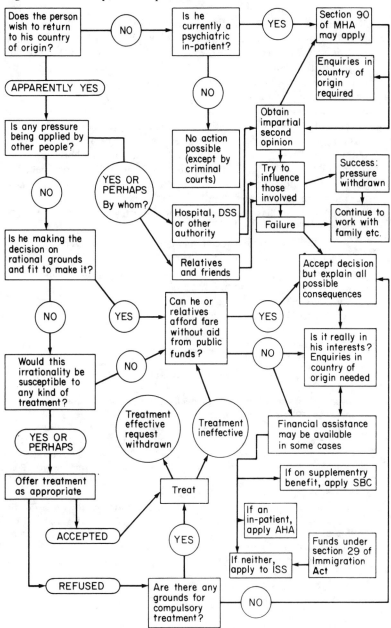

Figure 23 (1)   Repatriation procedure

places were really so idyllic the immigrant would not have come to Britain in the first place.

Repatriation, which may seem to be an obvious solution to the problems of some immigrants (whether psychiatric patients or not), is not, in practice, an easy option. Careful consideration is necessary before it is recommended, bearing in mind that the situation in the receiving country may be a lot less satisfactory than it appears from a distance and that many who do go back, subsequently wish they had not done so and may be unable to return to Britain. Those who wish to dispose of troublesome problems by sending them abroad should be carefully scrutinized for ulterior motives, and this applies equally to family and friends on the one hand, and hospital authorities on the other. For psychiatric conditions that are amenable to treatment and have a good short-term prognosis, it is nearly always better to arrange treatment in this country and allow the patient to make his own decisions after he has recovered. The long-term prospects must then be explained to him or his relatives.

Once the decision has been made to recommend repatriation, if assistance is required from public funds a great deal of time and effort may be needed to obtain this from the appropriate source. The process is likely to take at least six months.

The principal steps which should be taken in considering repatriation are set out schematically in Figure 23 (1).

NOTES

1 Statement of changes in Immigration Rules, HMSO 394 February 1980. Paras 56/7.
2 This is demonstrated by figures provided by the Bradford Education Department. In 1978 the department registered 699 children (ages 5-18) arriving from India, Pakistan or Bangla Desh. Three hundred and forty-five of those (49 per cent) were returning from visits, having been born in Britain (246) or lived here previously (99). Several had made more than one such visit (Annual report on the Education of Children of parents from the New Commonwealth and Pakistan, Appendix 5. Bradford Metropolitan Council, November 1978).
3 Lord Avebury, letter to Interdepartmental Committee on the Review of the Mental Health Act 1959. (Personal communication, 25.11.76).
4 Information provided by Supplementary Benefits Commission 1977. (Personal communication).
5 Information provided by ISS 1980. (Personal communication.)

24

Race, Law, and Psychiatry

The interface between law and psychiatry is always a difficult area, and the interaction of law and 'race' is notoriously acrimonious. Put the three together and we have an explosive mixture indeed. The practitioner who gets into this arena can safely assume that whatever he does will be criticized. Some representatives of the law have a stereotype of psychiatrists (and social workers) as 'soft option' people, whose aim is to help criminals to avoid their just deserts — 'bleeding hearts' who obfuscate simple issues of right and wrong by complicated psychologizing. On the other hand the civil-liberties lobby regard the psychiatrist as an agent of social control in the service of a repressive establishment, and mental hospitals as places where innocent victims are locked up and have harmful treatments inflicted on them simply because they do not conform to the wishes of society. To the practitioner, both these stereotypes probably seem ridiculous: but on reflection they are both seen to contain just enough truth to be uncomfortable. We must not be surprised to encounter them, and when 'race' is an additional factor we must tread with unusual care to avoid strengthening them: because in that case the 'repressive establishment' is, of course, the dominant (white) society, and the 'complicated psychologizing' can become very complicated indeed.

We are not concerned in this chapter with the question whether certain ethnic minorities commit more (or less) crime or simply get arrested more (or less) frequently (Bottoms 1973; McCulloch, Smith and Batta 1974, 1975). We may assume that every section of the population contains a few people who knowingly break the law, and that most crimes that are committed have no 'psychiatric' motivation. Leaving those aside, we have a problem when a person breaks the law and at the same time behaves in ways which raise the question of mental illness. The psychiatrist may then be called upon to tell the court whether or not the offender is mentally ill.

Consider the case of a youth whose unconstructive and objectionable behaviour is causing concern to his parents and teachers, so they send him to see a psychiatrist. He is not very co-operative, but the practitioner learns enough to realize that the youth is unhappy and confused. The identity doubts and capricious moods of adolescence are being exacerbated, perhaps (if he is of an ethnic minority background) by racial stigmatization, cultural ambiguity, and the inability of his parents to comprehend his world. The practitioner does not ask himself whether or not this youth is 'ill'. He could do with some help in sorting himself out, if help could be offered in a way he would accept. But what will be the effects on this youth if he is accepted as a patient? His 'treatment' will be very little different from what would be provided by a Youth Worker or some other practitioner. They would probably call it 'counselling', but if it is done by a psychiatrist it will inevitably be called 'psychiatric treatment', and because it takes place in a medical setting his parents and teachers will inevitably regard him as 'ill'. More importantly, the subject himself may come to regard his behaviour as 'illness', and that has all sorts of possible consequences, one of which is 'therefore I can't help it'. Bearing this in mind, it may be wiser not to go on seeing this patient, but refer him to some other agency.

Now suppose that six months later the same youth has broken the law, and the psychiatrist is asked to prepare a report for use in court. There are certain things which should be said about his background and his emotional conflicts, and they may influence the court's view of the offence and affect the sentence which is given. If the psychiatrist believes that simple punishment is likely to make matters worse instead of better, he will be tempted to say that what this youth needs is treatment; and if the psychiatrist is prepared to offer treatment, and the offence was not a major one, the court may well accept the suggestion. Everyone should now be happy.

But should they be? What has actually happened? Six months earlier it seemed wiser not to enrol this youth as a psychiatric patient because that would define him as 'ill'. Now here we are in court offering 'treatment'. He committed an offence, but nothing else has changed in the meantime. Is he ill or isn't he? Was he ill before or wasn't he? Mental illness seems to be a matter of convenience. The psychiatrist who gets himself into this sort of muddle exposes himself to the scorn of any legal mind, or indeed any logical mind. All this could have happened (and frequently does) whatever the ethnicity of the offender. But if the youth was a member of an ethnic minority there may be a barrage of criticism from another direction. 'Victimization!' these voices will cry. 'This boy has been oppressed, stigmatized, rejected because he is black. His behaviour is a protest and now you have the nerve to add to his troubles by labelling him as mentally ill, scapegoating him even more!' The hapless psychiatrist may want to explain that he was only trying to be helpful, but his stern-faced critics ask if he really believes that labelling people as 'ill' is helpful. References to Russian dissidents, South Africa, colonial exploitation, and racism get into the argument, until eventually the psychiatrist retreats, bemused and angry, wishing he had never got involved in the case.

The only way to avoid this is to think very clearly about what we are trying to say and are competent to say. The first thing the court wants to know from the practitioner is: 'Is there any reason to treat this offence differently from the way we usually treat offences of this kind?' If we think there is, it might be for two different reasons.

In a case of psychosis, the psychiatrist can usually speak with some authority. For example, a paranoid schizophrenic who assaulted a bystander because be believed himself to be under attack, or a depressed person who set fire to his house lest its evil influence pollute the world, may be thought to be, at the time, unaware of the nature and consequences of the act. In that case, the court will more often than not accept the suggestion that he be placed under psychiatric care. Generally, this will be a person who ought to have been receiving psychiatric care in any case, even if no crime had been committed.

If the psychiatrist believes that the offender was aware of the nature and consequences of his act, he must say so just as clearly, and leave it to the court to deal with the offence as it thinks best. He might have nothing more to say, but on the other hand he might think it right to draw the attention of the court to certain matters which seem to him to have a bearing on the offence. If so, this forms a different part of his report, in which he adopts an explanatory rather than an authoritative role and suggests respectfully that the court might have these points in mind in determining sentence. These are not statements about criminal responsibility, or the presence or absence of illness; they are psychological and social factors which can be taken into account. In the case described above, it is under this heading that the youth's emotional conflicts should have been mentioned.

DELUSIONS AND CRIMINAL RESPONSIBILITY

The issue of criminal responsibility is usually in question in cases of psychosis and severe mental handicap. Psychological and social factors can be taken into account in a much wider field. In the diagnosis of psychosis, loss of contact with reality and the presence of delusions can be a critical factor, so in this context we have to be even more precise than usual in our definition of delusion. We may think that a Jehovah's

Witness is misguided in his attitude to blood transfusions, or we may disagree with a Catholic about contraception, but we do not lock them up for their beliefs, nor inflict psychiatric treatment on them. The same should apply to the Muslim, or the Rastafarian, or the peasant whose world is peopled by unseen spirits, or the political extremist. Their beliefs, and actions arising from them, may make life difficult for the person and tax the tolerance of society in general, but they are not in themselves evidence of a need for psychiatric treatment. By the same token if such a person breaks the law, even if his crime is related to those beliefs, the psychiatrist should not be brought into it — at least, not on the criminal responsibility issue. If a devout Muslim father is offended by the thought of his teenage daughter mixing with boys, and restricts her activity to an extent which society in general considers unreasonable, there is no reason for a psychiatrist to be brought in at all, but if he is, he can only adopt a counselling or advisory role. Now if the father is prosecuted for keeping his daughter away from school, there is still no reason for the psychiatrist to become involved, but if he is, his role must still be only advisory: he can draw the attention of the court to the social and cultural background, but that is all.

A belief which, in one person, is a delusion (and therefore relevant to the question of mental disorder, and to the issue of criminal responsibility), may not be a delusion in somebody else. Suppose that a person accused of stealing other people's property defended himself on the grounds that all the fruits of the earth belong to God and cannot therefore be owned by an individual. The court could probably be persuaded quite easily to regard this defendant as mentally ill, and not capable of forming criminal intent. In most cases that would probably be a correct interpretation, but if the defendant were a member of a religious sect in which that belief was generally accepted, it would not be a delusion — so unless there were some other evidence of mental disorder the psychiatrist would not be able to intervene (except in his explanatory role). This may seem hard on the defendant who would otherwise have had a psychiatric defence, but it is essential to stick to the principle, because if we do not we are equating minority beliefs with madness, and in the long run that is a greater injustice.

An example from the author's own experience concerns a young man who had suffered from abdominal pain for some years, and who finally became convinced that his pain was the result of black magic. He believed that his former girl-friend had put a curse on him, and the only way he thought it could be stopped was to kill her, and that is what he did. He was duly charged with murder. Was he criminally responsible? His belief was certainly false (as he himself discovered when his pains continued unabated after her death), but was it a delusion?

In most people in Britain such a belief would be a delusion, but this event actually occurred in a Caribbean island where belief in black magic is commonplace. His explanation of his pain would have been shared — indeed, was shared — by the majority of his friends. It was not evidence of mental illness. Since on that island murder still carries the death penalty, the issue of his criminal responsibility was literally a life-and-death issue. Fortunately, in this case there were other criteria on which to make a diagnosis of psychosis.

DISSOCIATED STATES AND PSYCHOGENIC PSYCHOSES

Hysterical fugues and states of genuine dissociation, in which a person might commit an offence and afterwards claim complete amnesia for what took place, pose a particular problem. Because these are basically psychogenic, and usually have some unconscious motivation that entitles us to regard them as hysterical, we tend to view them a little differently from those conditions (e.g. schizophrenia or manic-depressive psychosis) which are at least partly 'biological' in aetiology. The following two cases are given at length because they exemplify this.

A woman who was born in rural Jamaica and came to Britain at the age of seventeen was referred to a psychiatrist eleven years later at her own request because of outbursts of unprovoked violence. The most recent of these had occurred at a wedding reception: she had suddenly become enraged, started shouting obscenities and smashing bottles and glasses, and had attacked her brother and some of the guests. She was assumed to be drunk and was forcibly taken home and put to bed, and she eventually slept. In fact she had drunk very little, and there were three previous episodes, only slightly less dramatic, which were in no way related to drink. On awakening afterwards she had, in each case, no memory of the events and she was embarrassed when told about them.

She later mentioned some other symptoms and in particular she spoke of seeing ghosts. These were three faceless figures, one of whom was female, which she had seen from time to time, often but not always at night, for as long as she could remember. Recently the female apparition had appeared more frequently, and had acquired an aura of menace. She felt that this ghost was influencing her against her will and was the cause of her behaviour. Asked if she thought she was 'possessed' by it she was evasive. There was no evidence of epilepsy or any other organic condition, and eventually she was given a diagnosis of schizophrenia and started treatment with phenothiazine drugs. If she had appeared in court at that time (charged with assault or criminal damage), no doubt the diagnosis of schizophrenia would have been used in her defence, and it would probably have been accepted as mitigation.

She defaulted from the clinic, but returned nine months later after a further similar episode. On this occasion she was seen by clinicians with some experience of Jamaican patients, and a different view was taken of her symptoms. Hallucination of ghosts ('duppies') is relatively commonplace in rural Jamaica and is of little or no psychiatric significance in itself. She was encouraged to talk about her feelings. Her mother, who had died the year before, was portrayed by her as an ideal figure with whom she had strong bonds — but that portrayal did not fit the facts. It became apparent despite her initial denials that she harboured many grievances against her family and also against the male sex in general. Altogether, there was plenty of material for a psychotherapeutic approach. She was told, in effect: 'We do not think you are suffering from schizophrenia, or any other form of madness, and we do not think you are posessed by any ghosts. We think you have a great deal of anger and frustration which you have been bottling up, and that is the cause of your behaviour'. She did not immediately agree about the bottled-up anger, but she said (with a smile) that she also did not think she was 'mad', and had opted out of treatment previously because she thought it was on the wrong lines and she did not like taking drugs. It was then put to her that if she was not 'mad', her outbursts of violence would not be excused on the grounds of madness, and in future she would be held responsible for them. When next seen, she said that this statement had been a great shock to her, but on reflection she had accepted it. She was never very co-operative with psychotherapy, and eventually ceased attending, but there were no further violent outbursts.

The second case, which did go to court, concerned a Pakistani village woman in her early thirties, who had left home several times for no apparent reason, turning up a few hours later in a state of distress, with no recollection of what had happened in the interim. The first such event occurred in Pakistan when she was in her teens. After she came to Britain at the age of twenty-three there were at least five repetitions. On one occasion she was arrested by railway police, having travelled to another city (apparently at random) with no ticket. Another time she stopped a patrolling police car and indicated that she had run away from her husband because he had beaten her — which was untrue. At all other times she was regarded as a stable and competent woman with no psychiatric problems and average intelligence. There were a lot of problems in the family. Her husband was lame from an injury and persistently unemployed though medically quite fit to work; most people regarded him as unreliable, evasive, and probably dishonest. The patient seemed to be the one who held the family together, but she voiced no criticism of her husband (except during the disturbed episodes).

One of her children was disabled following an injury in infancy for which she might have been (or might have been accused of being) responsible. She never spoke about this, and seemed to care for the child and the rest of the family with concern and affection.

In four of these 'runaway' episodes she was examined psychiatrically at the time or soon afterwards. Each time she was agitated and depressed, unable to speak coherently, and seemingly disorientated. Each time she recovered within hours, stating that she was now quite well and wanted to go home to look after her family, and protested vehemently if this was not permitted. She seemed genuinely perplexed when told what she had done during the period of amnesia. This patient spent many months in hospital, and she was examined by several psychiatrists, including two forensic experts and two Urdu-speaking consultants.

The majority opinion was that her amnesic episodes were hysterical fugues, presumably a manifestation of intolerable conflict of which she herself was genuinely unaware because of a very efficient mechanism of internal repression. When she acted in that way she was in a dissociated state which was cut off from everyday consciousness. It proved impossible to confirm this diagnosis, but if we assume it to be correct for the purposes of the present discussion, the point which concerns us is: can she be held fully responsible for actions committed in that state? This is no academic question, because in one of the episodes (the one which brought her to psychiatric attention) she got up early one morning while the rest of the family were still sleeping and walked off into the city *having first poured paraffin on some bedding and set it on fire*. Fortunately one of the children was awakened by the smell of burning and the fire was extinguished. She was charged with arson, and narrowly escaped a charge of attempted murder.

The court's dilemma was simple. If when starting the fire she was aware of the nature and consequences of that act she was manifestly a very wicked and dangerous woman who ought to be imprisoned for a long time. But her behaviour at all other times was not that of a wicked woman. But could the court accept hysteria as a defence?

In the end the court accepted the evidence of a psychiatrist (not the author) that at the time of the offence she had been psychotic, but had since recovered. She was placed on probation with a condition that she receive psychiatric treatment as and when required. This outcome may be thought rather questionable, but it is difficult to see how the interests of justice would have been served better by any other verdict or sentence.

In both these two cases the psychiatric assessment was that the behaviour was motivated, but unconsciously motivated. That need not alter our response to the crucial question which is: were they, at the material time, aware of the nature and consequences of their acts, and that the acts were wrong? Different practitioners might express different views on that, but the question can be considered in its own right, without bringing in diagnostic labels such as 'hysteria' which serve only to confuse the issue and are, in any case, speculations about aetiology rather than descriptions of mental state. Because of the prevalence of psychogenic psychoses and dissociated states in other cultures, and their rarity in British clinical practice generally, cases of this kind are quite likely to pose unfamiliar problems for British practitioners and the need for clarity of thought is the greater.

DELIBERATELY INDUCED DISSOCIATION

When the state of dissociation is deliberately induced by drugs, dancing, ritual or other procedure specifically designed for that purpose (see Chapter 12) is the subject legally responsible for actions taken while in that state? Could 'Possession' be used as a defence in law? It seems likely that a court would take the same view as is taken with alcohol intoxication. An extremely intoxicated person who commits an offence is held to be legally responsible because it is assumed that when he took the decision to become intoxicated he was aware of the possible consequences of doing so.

FITNESS TO PLEAD

A person charged with an offence may be regarded as unfit to plead if he or she is unable to conduct a defence and give instructions to defending counsel or is unable to follow proceedings in court. This is a humane dispensation for use in cases of severe mental or physical illness, or severe mental retardation, or when the defendant is deaf and dumb, when normal court procedure would be a travesty of justice. The law does not state that unfitness to plead is limited to those conditions, though it is usually the case in practice. To what extent should linguistic and cultural problems be taken into consideration in determining fitness to plead? Suppose a person who speaks no English, is of low intelligence and no education, has been in Britain only a short time and has committed a petty offence. He stands in court bemused, frightened, and bereft of all power of thought; it is quite obvious that he is unable to conduct a defence or follow court proceedings. His own counsel might wonder if he was fit to plead, or the question might be raised by the prosecution or from the bench. Psychiatric examination would then be requested.

Because the criteria of fitness to plead are different from, and in some ways less rigorous than, the criteria of criminal responsibility, there is no legal reason why linguistic and cultural factors should not be taken into account. But there is a hidden catch. If the plea is accepted, whatever the reasons for the unfitness, it is an automatic consequence that the accused will be admitted to a mental hospital and detained there compulsorily. His case has not been heard, so his guilt has not been established, let alone his sanity: yet he is locked up.

In practice, therefore, unless there is demonstrable and treatable mental disorder, it is customary to pretend that the accused is fit to plead even when he manifestly is not. This is quite unsatisfactory, but the alternative is worse, not only for the person who gets locked up, but for the hospital which has to accommodate him, and ultimately for society because compulsory psychiatric treatment ought to be based on strict clinical criteria and anything else is a corruption of psychiatry in any country. Therefore, as long as the finding of 'unfit to plead' has this automatic consequence, unless a person is in need of psychiatric care it does him no service to suggest that he is unfit to plead even though he has only the faintest idea of what is happening.

This example, like the very first one, illustrates the basic dilemma of the transcultural psychiatrist. There may well be reasons why a member of an ethnic minority ought to be dealt with by a court (that is to say, by society) slightly differently from someone else who has behaved in the same way, and in the interests of justice the court should be made aware of the differences. The psychiatrist may be the only person in a position to do that, but in coming forward to make those points the psychiatrist inevitably brings into the courtroom the implicit associations of 'mental illness'. By saying, 'society should take account of cultural diversity — I say this speaking as a psychiatrist' he runs the risk of being thought to say that cultural diversity is a psychiatric matter, though the message he wanted to put across might have been the exact opposite.

Improvement

25

Prevention: Health Education

So far, we have focused attention on what some members of ethnic minorities believe and how they behave, not what they *should* believe or how they *should* behave: we have tried to stick to the psychiatrist's role as an *enabler* who attempts to reveal what the issues are so that people can make their own decisions about them. The principle of cultural relativism demands that we refrain from the assumption that our own ethnocentric values are always the best. In this final Part we shall try to stick to the same approach, and point out not *what* changes should be made, but *how* changes can be made: looking first at the client and second at the practitioner.

There are people whose professional task is Health Education. They have two jobs to do: (1) teaching members of the public how to avoid illness, cope themselves with minor illness, and use the Health Service effectively when they need it; (2) teaching those employed in the Health Service how to make their service available and acceptable to the public they serve.

EDUCATING THE PUBLIC

Health Educators have a rather bossy, paternalistic image. They tell people not to do things that they enjoy like smoking, drinking alcohol, overeating, and travelling without seat belts. They are like Auntie who knows best what is good for us. This may be acceptable for simple issues like cleaning teeth but in the field of mental health, if we are considering cultural compromises and adaptation to new situations, didactic instruction obviously will not do.

There is a need for those members of ethnic minorities who have recently arrived in Britain, especially if they have moved from a rural to an urban environment, to be given instruction in certain basic health matters.[1] There is also a need to find out what their attitudes are to the statutory health services, and discover any problems which they may have in utilizing them properly.

A pilot study carried out by Bradford Health Education Unit found that Asian women tended to be late in booking at antenatal clinics, and even those patients who had one or more previous pregnancies in Bradford showed no consistent tendency to book earlier on second and subsequent occasions (Horne 1978). This was taken to indicate that educational endeavours by the clinic staff and the health education daprtment were not having much effect. Reasons for late booking were thought to include: (1) pregnancy is not seen as a 'disease' requiring medical attention: and (2) some of the clinic procedures (examination by a male doctor, blood sampling) were alarming or culturally offensive. The figures for low birth weight, stillbirth, and baby deaths in the neonatal and post-natal periods were consistently higher for Asian than for non-Asian births, sometimes by a factor of two or more, and comparing the Bradford statistics for twelve years up to 1978 showed no consistent improvement in these rates. The figures for severe subnormality among the Bradford-born children of Asian parents, were three times the non-Asian rate (Rowell and Rack 1979). Congenital deafness also occurs more frequently among Asian children (Hoyle, personal communication). We cannot be sure that these differences are all due to poor antenatal care. Protein deficiency during pregnancy due to Unani concepts of 'hot' and 'cold' foods, and lead poisoning due to use of Kushtay and Surmas (see Chapter 19) may play a part. Research is needed in these areas, but *in the meantime* since no woman wishes to jeopardize her pregnancy or her child there is a need for education. However, health education will be ineffective as long as it fails to take cultural beliefs into account.

In considering mental rather than physical health the issues are less clear-cut, and it is usually impossible to make simple cause-and-effect connections. Nonetheless, there are points which can be made about areas of stress that the person concerned, or the family, or the whole community have failed to recognize, and there is certainly a need for more information about appropriate sources of help. In trying to get these messages across we can draw on the experience of technical aid workers in developing countries. Foster (1973) describes many examples of educational and aid programmes that have gone wrong, and a few that have gone right, and suggests some useful ground rules. Rogers and Shoemaker (1974) proposed a theory of communication of innovation, and set up a model which has been adapted to health education by Tones (1977). According to this model, innovations that are introduced into a community from outside are more likely to be accepted if they are perceived by the community to be:

(1) advantageous
(2) compatible with existing practices
(3) simple
(4) trialable
(5) observable.

Roger's and Shoemaker's model depends on the identification of two sets of key figures, respectively called *Change Agents* and *Opinion Leaders*. The model is depicted schematically in Figure 25 (1).

Figure 25 (1) A model for the communication of innovation

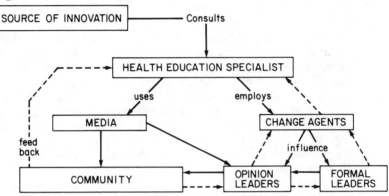

Opinion leaders, as the name indicates, are those in the community who influence others with greater than average frequency. They have referent or charismatic authority, whether or not they hold any formal leadership role. They are usually of relatively high social status, great social participation and accessibility, and are more exposed to the media.

An opinion leader may be monomorphic i.e. have a valued opinion on one subject only, or polymorphic. His or her authority may or may not be derived from technical competence. He or she must not be so traditional as to oppose all change, but on the other hand in order to retain authority, a leader must conform more or less to prevailing social norms. Innovativeness is a deviant activity by which social status is jeopardised, so it can only be practiced up to a point — not too much change at one time. In an Asian community, polymorphic opinion leaders are usually the men, especially the senior men in a family, backed up by the authority of the Mullah or Imam. In matters of pregnancy, childbirth, and child care, senior women (usually the mother-in-law) claim a monomorphic authority, and in health matters generally this is backed by the greater authority of the Hakim or Vaid. In Caribbean culture senior women have a more polymorphic authority, and other important opinion leaders include Obeah practitioners and in a more general sense the Pastors of Ministers of the 'Black' Churches. Rogers and Shoemaker suggest that innovations cannot be successfully introduced if these opinion leaders are 'by-passed', and if that is the case there is little point in giving health education lessons to (for example) pregnant women unless their mothers or mothers-in-law are also included.

Change Agents (see Figure 25 (1)) function as the intermediaries between the expert and the opinion leaders, and they must, therefore, be accessible and acceptable to both. They must have a clear understanding of the information which is to be imparted, and an equally clear and empathic understanding of the people to whom they impart it. They have, in fact, the characteristics that we have already described as desirable in an interpreter, and the same training needs. In practice, if we are considering a community or a family which is linguistically or culturally isolated from the rest of society, the change agent is anyone who has the ability of 'penetrate' that community and has succeeded in doing so. He or she may be a social worker, health visitor, community nurse or other health-care professional; or a home tutor, teacher, or neighbour who would not normally feel competent to advise on health matters. Under other circumstances, we are accustomed to calling in a different specialist to deal with questions outside our own narrow field of competence, but that cannot always be done in this case. The person who is accepted, who has rapport and has gained personal authority as an adviser in one sphere, finds that that authority is not instantly transferable. When it becomes apparent that there is no point in directing an enquiry elsewhere because the client will not go elsewhere, or is unlikely to explain the matter adequately if he does, the person who has the access must either ignore the problem or do the best he can, seeking what guidance he can get in the meantime. Thus the home tutor may find herself acting (apprehensively) as a 'barefoot' nurse, doctor, social worker, careers adviser, solicitor, and psychiatrist. This is not a satisfactory situation but it is what happens. The task of the expert, therefore, is to provide such a person with the information and advice which is needed, as and when it is needed, and support them in doing the job which, under other circumstances, he would expect to undertake himself. A cross-discipline resource centre in every area, with open access to all workers in the field, would provide invaluable back-up to people in this position. It could be located at a teaching hospital or existing specialist unit, but if these are not available the Health Education Unit seems an appropriate place.

EDUCATING THE PROFESSIONALS

The other, and equally important, task in health education is the education of professional workers and administrators in the health service, to give them more insight into the culture patterns and current problems of the various minority groups in their districts, and to point out how these affect health and behaviour. Fortunately, many hospital staff, health visitors, community nurses, and others recognize their need for knowledge and are keen to acquire it. This welcome trend has gathered momentum in recent years, and there have been many in-service training courses, day seminars, and study days, frequently over-subscribed. Participants have said later:

'My sympathy has increased. I was able to show sympathy for a man who came late for an appointment because he had been to pray.'

'The most useful thing was the explanation of the naming system, We have problems getting the names the right way round.'

'After the sessions I went back and asked patients about their cultures. It helped to establish a rapport.'

'I can identify more with the difficulties women in particular have to put up with ...'

(West Yorkshire Language Link 1978)

Bearing in mind that 'mental illness' is not the sole prerogative of mental health specialists, a large part of the syllabus of such courses would be of equal value to practitioners in other disciplines, and in view of the point made earlier about practitioners acting as 'barefoot' advisers outside their own speciality, there would seem to be every advantage in establishing such training on a multidisciplinary basis. There is no virtue in limiting it to people with professional or official status − on the contrary, a welcome can be extended to anyone with a legitimate interest in the subject. This has been the practice for many years at the Transcultural Psychiatry Unit at Bradford (see Appendix 4).

NOTE

1 Much of the material in this chapter is derived from a previous article: 'Health Education needs of a Minority Ethnic Group' (Rowell and Rack 1979). I am indebted to my co-author Mrs V. Rowell for permission to refer to it again here.

26

Working Across Cultures

The opening pages of this book depicted a meeting between two people. One, whom we called the client, had come to seek some kind of help which he was entitled to expect the other, the practitioner, to provide. The practitioner (it was assumed) wanted to do as good a professional job for this client as he or she would do for any other; but found himself, or herself, hampered by unfamiliar factors which we have designated 'cultural'.

This opening scene has been implicit in all that has followed. It is to that practitioner (whatever his field of work) that this book was primarily addressed, and its aims will have been fulfilled if, having worked through the intervening chapters, the practitioner now feels just a little less baffled by his task.

But what a grotesquely unbalanced scene it is! The practitioner is depicted as an intelligent, skilful, wise, compassionate, high-status member of the dominant (white) culture. The representative of the ethnic minority is cast in the supplicant role: it is his cultural peculiarities, his unfortunate experiences, his failure of adaptation that cause the problems. He is the one seeking help, and he adds to the work-load of the helper by his failure to conform to the rules of the situation. The helper has no intention of altering the rules, but is sufficiently generous to relax them just a little to enable the client to creep within, and learn how to conform better in future. It is a portrait of paternalism, the white man's burden all over again. And yet, like it or not, it reflects the realities of the present situation. The majority of the help-givers are indigenous and white. So, for that matter, are most of their clients. The ones who are not are the exceptions — that is inherent in the word 'minority'. The structures of society are set up by the majority (or a dominant elite within it) and in any society which even professes democracy they are set up with the needs of the majority in mind. This is presumably what those sociologists mean who define 'minority group' only in terms of disadvantage or oppression. The Scots in England are in a minority, but they are not a minority *group* because they do not experience adverse treatment as a group — there are Scots in every stratum of society. Can we envisage a time when the same will be true of Britons of Caribbean, Indo-Pakistani, or Indo-Chinese ancestry? The optimistic answer is yes, and we should work towards it. But by the time we get there, those groups will have ceased to be groups, they will have become part of the majority. To say that power lies with the majority is a truism that leads nowhere: the question is, how is that power used? To complain that the help-givers (the practitioners) are in a dominant position *vis-à-vis* their clients is pointless: they are on the giving rather than the receiving end of the transaction because that is what they are there for, that is their function in that situation. To complain that most practitioners belong to the majority culture is equally pointless. For one thing it is not strictly true (there are a great many Asian doctors, and the question why not all Asian patients choose to consult them has been mentioned already and will be again) but we can complete our sociological truisms by observing that once a member of a minority group gets into a practitioner role he acts as an agent for the structure/society as a whole, and has become (in his professional activities) a member of the majority. If our portrait of the paternalistic practitioner and the supplicant client gives offence, so be it: there is nothing we can do about it. Practitioners are not politicians, it is not our task to change society. We have to operate as best we can in the here and now.

Yet that is not quite true, because after all we do have quite a lot to do with policy. There are two things we can do; one alternative is to tell the client to go away. If he wishes to maintain his cultural separateness, let him set up his own structures and systems to solve his own problems in his own way. Let him use Obeah and Hakims and develop his own community-based social and welfare services — in fact because he is saving us money by not using our service, we will make funds available for him for the purpose.

As soon as we start to think this through, we see where it leads. There is a word for separate development, and it is *apartheid*. There are groups in Britain who choose to do their own thing and live in parallel with the main society but separate from it. Gypsies, for example, avoid the National Health Service and most other services as much as possible, but this is their choice — they are not refused admission. Because no ethnic minority can command financial resources to match those of the State, any parallel development would remain impoverished unless it were subsidized — and in subsidizing it we are back to paternalism. 'Separate but Equal' makes a fine slogan, but the reality would be either separate and unequal, or equal and therefore not separate.

If we reject the idea of separateness our second alternative is to accept the idea of difference, and to do so not grudgingly but gladly. This ought not to be too difficult on a personal level, since the practitioner is accustomed to treating individuals on the basis of their personal requirements. Every doctor knows that influenza in a healthy schoolboy is different from influenza in a debilitated old lady living alone, and he tailors his treatment accordingly. The practitioner's work would be extremely dull and mundane if his clients were all the same. There ought not to be any difficulties at a policy-making level either. In a South Coast resort with a large retirement population, more resources must be allocated to geriatric provision; in a new town with a high birthrate, emphasis must be on maternity and child welfare. There is nothing revolutionary in suggesting that a district with a large ethnic minority population should find out what special needs they have, and adapt its services accordingly. Reluctance to do so may be due to prejudice — these people 'don't matter' enough — or it may be due to fear of the word discrimination.

Statements like 'I treat everyone the same whoever they may be' are just silly. If it is the case that children to whom English is a second language require extra coaching at school; or that women accustomed to the support of the extended family feel deprived and miserable if it is withdrawn; or that some people have experienced police brutality (whether in Nazi Germany, Uganda, or Brixton) and are sensitized to expect it; or that a particular medicine or diet is culturally unaccept-able, then failure to take these differences into account is itself a kind of adverse discrimination. To treat a Sikh as if he were not a Sikh is unproductive if he is determined to remain a Sikh. The implication is that everyone who comes to live in Britain should make haste to become British, and that is a theoretical view attractive only to people who are ignorant of practical and psychological realities. For the practitioner, dealing with real and immediate issues, the only choice is between recognizing differences in order to do his job well, or failing to recognize them and doing it badly.

Having decided to acknowledge the existence of differences, we must guard against the danger of stereotyping. I know two Nigerian students and they are both . . . so I assume that all Nigerian students are . . . and probably all Nigerians . . . and maybe all Africans (if I am not acquainted with any others). All the Bengalis I have met were . . . so I make certain assumptions or prejudgments about the next one I meet. A policeman who sees a well dressed white man running along the pavement in Oxford Street sees a man trying to catch a bus: if he sees a black youth running he sees (if he is prejudiced) a mugger running from the scene of a crime. That is what he *sees*: it is not a matter of logical thought or deduction, it is a matter of perception, based on the pre-conceived stereotype in that policeman's mind. We cannot do without stereotypes. We have not been able to avoid them in this book. Any student who sets out to learn a new subject is obliged to structure his material, to formulate categories and rules and generalizations in order to make sense of the incoming data that would otherwise remain disparate and unlearnable. We are not wrong if we say: 'According to my information so far, West Indians are . . .'. But we are wrong if we say (or unconsciously assume): 'Therefore all West Indians are . . .' — and dangerously wrong, because we shall attribute those characteristics to the next West Indian we meet, without waiting for evidence that might well show that he is, in fact, quite different. The temptation is pervasive because the process of categorization is such a useful tool to us in making sense of our environment. When a doctor is able to say that a patient has or does not have pneumonia he feels more able to control the situation, because 'pneumonia' is a category about which he can make certain predictions and treatment-decisions; but the experienced doctor does not expect every case of pneumonia to conform to his model, he expects some of his predictions to be wrong, and he does not attribute every aspect of the patient's behaviour to his pneumonia. In the process of making sense of new data, whether it be a new patient or a new culture, categorization is an important part of the process, but it is not as important as accurate observation, logical deduction, receptivity to contradictory evidence, and recognition of the limits of one's present knowledge. The danger is that categorization and stereotyping may take the place of those other activities. We all fall into this error and need colleagues who will shout when they catch us at it.

The practitioner who takes seriously his commitment to clients from other cultures must make the effort to familiarize himself with the cultures in question, and not simply the 'nuts and bolts' of the way people live, but the beliefs and value systems underlying that behaviour. A certain amount of this can be learned from books, but not everything, as local cultures are constantly developing. Knowledge of the village customs of a part of Pakistan is only a limited guide to the culture adopted by people from that area when they have lived some years in a British city, and even the descriptions available of minority groups in Britain are only accurate for the group described, and at the time of writing. There is no real alternative to getting out of the clinic or office, to meet people and ask questions.

That should not prove too difficult, given a modicum of initiative and sensitivity. As a general rule, any group of people who have a culture that matters to them, to which they adhere even when it is not easy to do so, are usually very pleased to receive enquiries from interested outsiders. Once they are convinced that the interest is genuine and without ulterior motives, they often respond with great warmth and friendliness (which may take the enquirer by surprise). Obviously anyone who treads clumsily, firing off a barrage of questions as if inspecting some exotic species in a menagerie, will get the reception he deserves. But if the questions are part of a genuine and friendly attempt to discover how the world looks through another person's eyes, without patronizing or pre-judgment, that is usually apparent and initial gaffes and gaucheries are usually forgiven.

There are exceptions to this. For example, those who have the culture and attitudes which were described in Chapter 4 under the general heading of 'peasants', may adopt the traditional peasant strategies for fending off outsiders. Anyone who has suffered repression under a totalitarian regime may have a fear — perhaps even a phobia — of being spied on. Some black people erect automatic barriers against all whites, and any white person who engages in conversation with any black person in Britain today should appreciate that blacks receive from white people a hundred snubs and belittlements daily. Not only the obviously disadvantaged immigrant but also the most articulate, self-possessed, and confident-seeming black person has had to cope with the stereotyping and scapegoating which white society inflicts indiscriminately on those with coloured skins. This being so, the enquirers should be prepared for a certain reaction which is perhaps best described as a 'thin-skinned defensiveness'. This may be apparent immediately or may be concealed. It takes time to establish mutual trust, and problems can reappear unexpectedly when disagreements arise even between friends who thought their relationship to be secure. For example, a black person reading this paragraph might be moved to retort that thin-skinned defensiveness is also found among whites — and go on to accuse the writer of creating another stereotype — the paranoid black. This is not intended, but it shows that in this discussion one cannot be too careful. Yet — one *can* be too careful. If there is to be real communication, we cannot afford to take refuge in bland platitudes, and the risk of misunderstanding must be accepted; it must not take us by surprise.

Indian and Pakistani families have an endearing habit of adopting outsiders into the family, ascribing names like 'Auntie' or 'sister'. The practitioner may find it a little disconcerting to be told 'You are my father', and this can happen whether the contact is a social or a professional one. Parekh (1974) has suggested that such usages are not simply a flattering mannerism, but indicate something about Indian culture. Because (Parekh suggests) Indian life revolves about family life, all relationships tend to be perceived in those terms. Within the family there are built-in and clearly understood roles and obligations between members: one has a certain relationship with one's wife's younger sister, or one's elder brother's wife, because of the structure of the group and irrespective of personal affection or antipathy. The links between members are — at least in part — lines of domination-subservience, protection-dependency, instruction-obedience, and so on. To place someone in a position on this sociogram is to define their interrelatedness to the whole group. No individual member has a relationship with someone outside the family that is his and his alone. The practitioner who finds himself 'adopted' into such a family is likely to feel pleased and grateful, and enjoy the (very genuine) warmth of his welcome. He is invited to attend family weddings, and expected to give and receive presents. It is all very pleasant; his own life is enriched by new experiences and friendships, and incidentally the cause of community relations is being advanced. There are not usually any problems in this situation, but problems can arise occasionally, particularly when the context of the relationship is professional rather than social. The social worker, home tutor, or health visitor has a limited role. He or she has particular professional obligations towards one member of the household and does not foresee a permanent relationship with the family when that obligation has been discharged. Agreeable though it may be to be accepted as a brother or sister, it is not an accurate perception — or at least it is not the social worker's own perception — of the political realities of the relationship. Disappointment and disillusionment may come if, for example, the social worker is asked to be an advocate on the family's behalf or use her supposed influence with 'authority' in some other department — requests that it is quite reasonable to make to a member of the family but which the social worker may feel are inappropriate. (The social worker has been used as an example here because the role of doctors, nurses, teachers, and some other practitioners is more clearly demarcated and understood. Social workers are something of a mystery.)

The practitioner who goes to the trouble of discovering the culture of a minority group (*any* different group) is rewarded by the satisfaction and sheer interest of seeing the world from a different standpoint, and is likely to find his or her own perceptions changed and sharpened. 'Travel broadens the mind' and gives one a different outlook on one's own life and one's ethnocentric values. This is not a passive process, however. There is work in it. If (for example) we perceive that in a certain culture women are subjected to male dominance, and given little opportunity to develop initiative or other characteristics which we think desirable, we find this offensive and dehumanizing — in a word, 'wrong'. If we take the trouble to learn about the culture as a totality, and recognize the value systems on which behaviour is based, and try to accept the culture in its own terms as an anthropologist does, we may find that the parts which we found offensive are inseparable from the whole, and the whole constitutes a viable system of social organization which we are not entitled to condemn. To take a different example: in many parts of the world family obligations and loyalties are a great deal stronger than they are now in Britain. An individual exists primarily as a member of a family, and tends to see himself in those terms. As long as he conforms to the accepted canons of behaviour he can count on the group to support him. Thus an Asian family in Britain may receive an arriving cousin or uncle, and house and feed him without question, however precarious its own financial position. At the same time, any member who offends against the mores of the group — for example an unmarried girl becoming pregnant — may be rejected and abandoned, literally turned out and forgotten.

The ruthlessness of this may seem surprising but it is only the obverse of the coin of group solidarity which in other ways seems admirable. The principle of total acceptance as long as the rules are obeyed depends on the principle of rejection if they are broken. You cannot have one without the other. Taken all round, is this system 'better' or 'worse' than our accustomed, *laissez-faire*, society? And in what sense can one use words like 'better' and 'worse'? Recognition of a different value system, which may not be accepted but cannot be repudiated either, brings with it the realization that one's own habitual values are culturally determined and one's own moral system is but one among many. The escape from ethnocentrism leads to a scrutiny of one's own unchallenged assumptions, and this is always an uncomfortable experience. In some respects the process is like a personal analysis or psychotherapy (Park 1928). It has some similar potential benefits for the individual, but also some similar pitfalls. The practitioner who previously handled moral decisions with confidence may now find himself adrift on a sea of uncertainty, anomic in a self-created marginality. Anyone who chooses to work across cultures must be prepared to experience this discomfort, and may require assistance in coping with it. It is potentially a valuable experience especially for those who work among immigrants, as it can provide some insight into the much greater degree of marginality and confusion which immigrants themselves experience, which underlie some of their emotional problems. To be utilized, however, the experience has to be brought forward into consciousness and accepted, not left as a half-conscious sense of vague uncertainty; otherwise the unconscious mind will find its own ways of escaping from the discomfort, and there are several possible positions, some of them false or unconstructive, into which to retreat.

For the 'marginal man' (Stoneqvist 1937; Park 1928) who finds himself spanning two cultures and at home in neither, the usual resolution of the problem is to make a conscious choice and identify with one or the other, or some third group, and hope to obtain acceptance and a sense of belonging in one group or another. The cross-cultural worker can, if he wishes, escape from his self-inflicted marginality in the same way, by opting for a primary identification with one culture only: if he has worked his way through to this position consciously and honestly he is by no means disqualified from continuing to work cross-culturally. Alternatively, he may opt to remain in a state of marginality, with all its attendant discomfort, believing that in that position he is best placed to help others to find their own resolutions. Both positions are tenable: false positions arise when the issue is not faced.

One such false position is *concealed ethnocentrism*. In this, the person pays lip-service to the principle of cultural relativism and takes pride in his open-mindedness, but maintains his own emotional security by using his original ethnocentric values as a secret refuge. Alternatively he may identify with the 'new' culture with an uncritical enthusiasm, refusing to accept any disparagement of even those aspects that people born into that culture find unsatisfactory. Or the one reaction may be, and probably often is, an overcompensation for the other. The white Englishman who waxes lyrical about the ancient wisdom of the East, or the pulsating vitality of Africa, or the moral virtues of Islam, should be viewed with some initial scepticism. He may be merely attracted by the stimulation of exotic novelties. We may suspect that his eager over-identification with a different culture reflects his failure to identify with his original group. He may be:

'The idiot who praises in enthusiastic tone
All centuries but this and every country but his own.'

(W. S. Gilbert)

We shall not be surprised if he moves on shortly to seek his own identity somewhere else.

For the white 'liberal' there is a particular temptation to become an advocate on behalf of oppressed minorities, as this is a morale-boosting and ego-boosting activity. As long as relatively few white people choose to step to and fro across cultural boundaries, those who do so can attain a special position. Members of the oppressed minority express their humble gratitude for his kindly interest. Those of the white peer group who feel vaguely guilty about race relations but are not doing anything about it themselves, join in the applause. The title of accredited expert is offered; and if it is accepted this introduces issues of self-esteem which can easily jeopardize any detachment about the actual extent of knowledge or value of the work. Loyalty to 'my' people leads to a compulsion to defend them against all criticism however mild or justified, an indiscriminate and sometimes strident advocacy. The white impassioned champion of coloured minorities is an increasingly familiar figure. He is important, and we shall not sneer at him, but we should keep the thought in our minds (and so should be), that race relations is a *good cause*, and good causes are tempting. As expressed by a contemporary playwright:

> '*Brian*: . . . You'd like a good fight, wouldn't you, George?
> *George*: Yes, I would. It's a scandal.
> *Brian*: It's a scandal. And they're hard to come by, aren't they? That's what you're missing and you'd enjoy it too much. Something really solid to get the life-giving adrenalin flowing.'
>
> (Alan Bennett, *Getting On*)

Among the fighters in this field there are many who have worked their way through the various processes already mentioned, who know what they are doing, and why; but it has to be said that the group also contains some who are unclear about their own motivations, and occupy false positions such as those described here. This is important, because it can invalidate good intentions. The thin-skinned defensiveness of black people puts them on the lookout for hypocrisy, patronizing paternalism, concealed or overcompensated hostility, latent ethnocentrism, or any other form of false posturing. They may see it when it is not there: they will certainly detect it sooner or later when it is. The situation has been reached where some militant black groups decline to accept support from so-called white liberals, because they suspect them to be working from false positions. This is an example of stereotyping, which is no more defensible than earlier examples: but it is sometimes correct.

The examples given so far have dealt with the adjustments to be made by members of the majority culture in working with members of minority groups, since that is the commonest situation. Similar problems arise when the position is reversed. The Indian doctor (for example) working in Britain is called upon to reconsider his attitudes and cultural values, and may require help in doing so and avoiding false positions. There is also another group of workers who experience conflicting value-systems, and these are the immigrants who have lived many years in Britain and are now joining the ranks of the practitioners as doctors, social workers, probation officers, or in a semi-professional capacity as interpreters. Such people are invaluable members of the therapeutic team, acting as intermediaries and able to get closer to the patient than any other member of the team: but they are able to occupy this intermediary position because they can straddle two cultures, and therefore they, too have the strengths and weaknesses inherent in marginality. This is strikingly illustrated by an unpublished experiment by Lipsedge in 1979 at a London hospital in which many of the nursing staff as well as many of the patients were of Caribbean origin. The (English) psychiatrists were sometimes unsure whether behaviour exhibited by such patients was culturally normal or evidence of psychosis, and they wished to enlist the help of the Caribbean nurses. They therefore produced a series of short case-descriptions and showed these 'borderline' vignettes to three groups of assessors. The group of English professionals expressed uncertainty but said they were prepared to believe that the things described could be culturally normal. The second group were Caribbean laymen with no psychiatric knowledge, and they accepted most of the descriptions as culturally normal. The third group were the psychiatric nurses of Caribbean origin, trained and qualified in Britain. They unhesitatingly classified most of the behaviour as psychotic! Lipsedge and his colleagues interpreted this to indicate that the psychiatrically trained and 'anglicized' nurses had repudiated their Caribbean norms (Lipsedge, personal communication). We might refer to this as the false position of 'overadaptation'. Where this exists, the therapeutic team obviously must not rely too heavily on the diagnostic acumen of such intermediaries. In Lipsedge's study it was possible to check because there was no actual language barrier, but this is much more difficult where all communication takes place through an interpreter and the interpreter's own value-systems are unclear.

There are an increasing number of young adults in Britain who were born here of immigrant parents, and have passed through the British education system and emerged with qualifications in sociology, politics, or some other field related to the general area we are discussing. Such people are, of course, invaluable: having their own experience of (for example) Indian family life and culture, they are in the best possible position to interpret one culture to the other, and are better qualified to do so than the present author. Having said that, however, we should not forget that they, too, straddle the boundaries and are not immune from the discomforts of marginality. However intelligent and well educated, they can have internal conflicts and contradictions which they may or may not have resolved.

It is clear from all this that working across cultures is a challenge. The difficulties are greatest when the values of the cultures are contradictory, and they are aggravated by the fact that one culture (the one to which most practitioners belong) is in a position of dominance over the other. It is significant that having started with the need to learn about customs and habits, and then recognized the need to understand the underlying moral values, we have arrived eventually at the need for the practitioner to scrutinize his own attitudes and prejudices. Facts can be learned from books. Cultural sensitivity comes only from exchanges in which attitudes are honestly challenged and honestly inspected.

It may be suggested that anyone who aspires to work across cultures should be carefully screened beforehand. This would be fine if we were setting out to train an elite corps of specialists, but the reality is that any practitioner, in any profession, may encounter a cross-culture situation from time to time, and it is only when the situation arises that the problems become apparent. For those who are frequently in such situations specialist training is certainly desirable, and it is becoming more widely available. In such training a good deal of time must be given to exploration by the trainee of his own beliefs and attitudes, (probably best undertaken in small-group seminars conducted along the lines of other sensitivity training groups). For the remainder, the generality of practitioners, is there a case for including more emphasis on cultures in the general curriculum?

Having conducted seminars on this subject with students for several years, the author believes firmly that there is such a case. It is illustrated by the student (usually the brightest one in the group) who says towards the end of the discussion — a great light dawning — 'But there are different cultures even in our own society!'. There are indeed: the practitioner who goes to work in South Wales, or the Yorkshire Dales, or the stockbroker belt in Surrey, will have to learn about the particular (and different) cultures of those places if he or she is to function effectively. Even where there are no immigrant communities a cultural perspective on behaviour is a valuable additional perspective. In theory it could be taught by reference to indigenous cultures alone: in practice students grasp the point more readily by starting with cultures in which the differences and their practical consequences are more obvious, and then (one hopes) applying this awareness across the board. The ethnic minorities in Britain are not just a nuisance group who place additional burdens on the system in general and the overworked practitioner in particular. If we are willing to listen, they will teach us a lot about ourselves.

Appendix 1
A Guide to Psychiatric Terminology and Classification

Non-medical practitioners are not expected to make psychiatric diagnoses, but they need to have some understanding of the various categories of mental illness if only to judge when specialist help is required. There are many different types of mental disorder, and discussion becomes confused if they are all lumped together as if they formed a single entity. The British classification system is not sacrosanct, and some of its deficiencies are discussed in chapters 10–15, but as it is in common use it provides a useful point of departure, and is described here in simplified form for the benefit of the non-specialist reader. The main categories are:

(A) Organic conditions
(B) Functional conditions
    (1) Psychoses
        (a) Affective disorders (Depression, Mania)
        (b) Schizophrenia
    (2) Neuroses.

The diagnostic process is depicted schematically in Figure 1.

The first question usually asked by any doctor is: 'When did it start?' If a person has been odd, eccentric, or difficult all his life, we shall probably not regard this as an illness but an attribute of personality, or *personality disorder*. Single-adjective descriptions are used as a kind of shorthand, but are better avoided, and it is better to describe the problem (e.g. 'Always had difficulty with close personal relationships'). The word 'Psychopathic' sounds as if it should have a precise meaning, but it has not. Some people with personality disorders can benefit from psychiatric treatment, but obviously behaviour that has been present lifelong is not easily altered. If the abnormality has not been present all along, we can ask: what was he like before this started? If there is a definite contrast, he was 'normal' before (at least, his quirks and oddities did not bother him or anyone else before) and has now become recognisably different and the difference is disadvantageous, then we are able to define his 'illness' in terms of the difference from his previous self. This also defines the task, which is (roughly speaking) to restore him to his former state.

The terms *acute* and *chronic* refer to the onset of the illness and its duration. An acute illness is of recent and sudden onset: a chronic one has been present for some time, (though the initial onset, when it started, might have been acute). They do not indicate severity.

ORGANIC CONDITIONS

The next step is usually to consider the possibility of a physical cause for the symptoms. Examples include damage to the brain by injury, infection, tumour, general metabolic disorders, fever or dehydration such as can occur with almost any serious illness, producing delirium: specific metabolic and endocrine disorders (e.g. diabetes, thyroid excess or deficiency); drug-induced disorders (e.g. alcohol intoxication); and degenerative disease of the brain, possibly due to arteriosclerosis, producing dementia. These conditions, in which the psychiatric symptoms have a demonstrable physical cause, are called *organic*. Once diagnosed, they are usually handed on for treatment to some other medical specialist.

FUNCTIONAL CONDITIONS

All other conditions, in which there is no demonstrable organic cause, are referred to as *functional* disorders. They are the main province of the psychiatrist and are divided into two main groups.

1. Psychoses

The psychoses are generally the more serious, and correspond most to the laymen's idea of madness.

(a) Affective disorders: the commonest is depression, called *depressive illness* or *endogenous depression* to distinguish it from the low feelings which everyone has in adversity (which if severe constitute *reactive depression*, to be considered later). The important feature of endogenous depression is that it comes on without sufficient external cause, and not only is mood affected but there much more generalized disruption of mental processes including loss of concentration and initiative, loss of enjoyment, feelings of guilt and self reproach, often leading to suicidal thoughts. A depressed patient may be *retarded* —

Figure 1 Schema of the diagnostic process

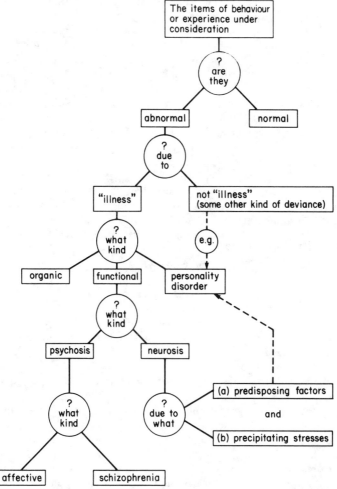

i.e. all mental processes and reactions are slowed down – or *agitated* – with accompanying tension and anxiety. The patient and relatives may attribute the depression to external causes, such as some recent change or misfortune, but the probability is that the patient has coped with such misfortunes in the past and would have done so again if in normal health. The stress is only a trigger factor. Probably many people have minor attacks of endogenous depression and recover spontaneously without seeking treatment. Treatment is by *antidepressant drugs* or electroplexy (ECT) and is nearly always effective in a few weeks. About one patient in three is likely to have a further attack some time in his life and some people have several.

Mania, or its less severe form *hypomania*, is the opposite state to depression. The hypomanic patient is overactive, restless, irrationally happy, full of vitality, overconfident, and likely to deny that there is anything wrong with him. His judgment is at fault, however, and he may behave in ways he will later regret — driving too fast, spending money extravagantly or giving it away, or saying and doing outrageous scandalizing things in public. He may even believe he has special, God-given powers. Hypomania is much less common than depression. It is usually fairly brief and recovers spontaneously but recovery is speeded up by appropriate treatment, which is by drugs. There is a tendency to recurrence, and a few people have attacks at frequent intervals.

A particular form of affective disorder is *manic-depressive psychosis* in which the patient is liable to have both depressive and manic episodes, sometimes alternating with clockwork regularity but more often irregularly. An important feature of all affective disorders is that they often affect people who, before becoming ill, were regarded as very competent, mentally robust, and stable individuals, and they recover completely.

(b) Schizophrenia: Whereas depression and mania are disorders primarily of mood or *feelings*, *schizophrenia* the other major functional psychosis, can be regarded as a disorder of the *thinking* processes. No-one really believes that schizophrenia is the name of one specific condition — it is a portmanteau term for several conditions which have features in common, for which separate causes will probably be discovered in time. It may come on insidiously, so that for years a person is regarded as being just a little eccentric; or acutely, with dramatic and bizarre manifestations. *Delusions* are a common feature of schizophrenia. A delusion is a false belief: for example, a patient may believe that people are following him about, communicating in code and plotting to kill him. These are *delusions of persecution*, called *paranoid delusions*. He might have grandiose delusions of supernatural powers, or having been chosen by a divine agency for a special mission. To rank as a delusion, a belief must be outside the range of normality for that person. This of course causes real difficulties in dealing with patients from different cultures. As well as thinking abnormal things a schizophrenic may be thinking *in an abnormal way*: his thought processes are disrupted so that ideas do not follow logically or consecutively but are juxtaposed or jump about by idiosyncratic associations which defy understanding. This kind of fragmentation is one sort of *schizophrenic thought disorder*. It is not always present or easily detected but when it occurs it is an

important diagnostic point not so much dependent on culture. *Halluci-nations* are also common in schizophrenia. A hallucination is a false perception – for example hearing voices when there are no voices.

Schizophrenia may occur at any age. Quite commonly it begins in early adult life. Unlike the affective disorders the prospects of spontaneous recovery without treatment are poor. Treatment is usually by drugs of the *phenothiazine* family (unfortunately misnamed 'tranquillizers') which should be supplemented by other, psychodynamic forms of therapy, but the latter are very little use on their own without drugs. Sometimes 100 per cent recovery is achieved, but usually rather less, and sometimes hardly any. Treatment relieves the symptoms, but apparently does not affect the underlying causes of them, so drugs have to be continued in a small 'maintenance' dose after recovery, because there is a strong probability of relapse if they are discontinued. In its severe forms schizophrenia is a grave and destructive disease and it is one of medicine's major unsolved problems. There are, however many people who have a few symptoms suggestive of schizophrenia without being greatly or permanently diabled. Such 'fringe' cases are more likely to be labelled schizophrenic by American psychiatrists than by British ones – which bedevils international and transcultural comparisons. There are also many people, correctly diagnosed as schizophrenic, leading normal or near-normal lives in the community because they continue to receive maintenance treatment.

The functional psychoses – that is, *endogenous depression*, *mania*, and the various varieties of *schizophrenia* – may be considered as diseases, comparable to diabetes or any other physical disease. Indeed, many psychiatrists believe that they *are* physical diseases, of which the underlying physical causes have not yet been discovered. There may well be biochemical abnormalities in the brain, but the evidence is not yet conclusive. There is little doubt, however, that treatment on medical lines is effective (not always perfectly) and such patients should receive medical care.

2. Neuroses

The neuroses should not be regarded as 'diseases' but as ways of reacting to stress. They are sometimes referred to as illnesses because the response is *maladaptive* i.e. it does not help to resolve the stressful situation and may indeed aggravate it. Everyone behaves neurotically sometimes. It is not surprising that the classification of neuroses is imprecise, since no two people react in the same way: but some generalization is possible.

Anxiety is a common human experience. As well as a subjective feeling of distressed apprehension, it includes physical components such as dry mouth, palpitations in the chest, abdominal discomfort, loose bowels, sweating, tension headaches, restlessness, and so on. These can all be accounted for by the release of adrenalin into the bloodstream, which is part of the organism's 'alerting mechanism' to meet threats. Anyone who is anxious may experience those sensations, and recognize them as stress reactions, and put up with them in the knowledge that they will go away once the stress is removed. A person suffering from the form of neurosis called an *anxiety state*, however, experiences these sensations continuously, which is very unpleasant. The cause of the anxiety may not be apparent to the sufferer, because it may be something he has chosen not to think about and face up to — or indeed *cannot* face up to, because the stress is so intolerable that it has to be *repressed*, kept out of consciousness altogether. In that case he is aware of the anxiety symptoms, but cannot account for them or control them, and is easily convinced that the thumping in his chest or the shortness of breath are due to heart disease or cancer. The physical reaction aggravates the anxiety, which in turn creates more physical tension and a vicious circle is established: an example of a *maladaptive response* to stress. It can happen that the tension, if continued, does eventually lead to structural damage in some part of the body: hence the association between stress and many other *psychosomatic disorders.*

Other examples of neuroses are reactive depression, hysteria, obsessional and phobic states.

Reactive depression differs from the endogenous depression considered already in that there is a reason for the reaction. It ranks as a neurotic illness if it becomes extreme, self-perpetuating, and chronic, when it may closely resemble endogenous depression, and require treatment along the same lines. In fact, it is quite common to decide that someone's depression is part-endogenous and part-reactive.

Hysteria. In colloquial speech 'hysteria' suggests an outpouring of unrestrained emotion, but psychiatrists use the term slightly differently. As applied to a personality, 'hysterical' usually indicates someone who is effusive and liable to over-react, but it also implies skill at manipulating people and situations for selfish ends. The hysterical personality seeks attention and solicits sympathy, often using persuasive techniques which amount to emotional blackmail. He or she does not act in this way with conscious deliberation, and will deny any such intention. The term is also applied to *symptoms*: an hysterical symptom being (initially) a disorder or disability for which there is no physical cause, but which is due to unconscious stress or unresolved conflict. The subject cannot face the conflict and represses it, but it reappears as an apparently unrelated physical complaint. He has no emotional problems (he says) and would feel fine if only his symptoms would go away. This kind of reaction is rather more common in subjects who have hysterical personalities — hence the overlapping terminology.

Phobic and obsessional states are other kinds of neurosis, characterized by the compulsive need to carry out certain actions or repeat certain thoughts (obsessions) or avoid certain things (phobias) although the subject realizes that there is no need to do so. Most people are phobic about something — spiders, worms, thunderstorms, high places — but are only disabled if the phobia interferes greatly with their activities. An *agaraphobic* patient, for example, may be unable to go out of doors unaccompanied without developing an acute attack of panic.

Because the neuroses are stress reactions it follows that treatment on 'medical' lines with drugs is unlikely to relieve the symptoms for long unless something is done about the causes of stress. This might be removing the stress, or assisting the patient to face up to it and resolve conflicts or otherwise come to terms with them.

It follows that in relation to neuroses and psychosomatic illness the process of psychiatric diagnosis is not complete until the stresses which are causing the symptoms have been made clear. Since the symptoms have often arisen because the patient is unable to face up to the underlying causes, the practitioner has to take the initiative in exploring likely problem areas, and may well encounter resistance from the patient in doing so. This is all part of the process called *psychotherapy*.

Psychoanalysis as devised by Freud, and the various modifications developed by his successors, are not greatly employed in Britain in their original forms, but Freudian concepts and insights enter into most types of psychotherapy. *Group therapy* and *family therapy* are forms of psychotherapy. Sometimes the maladaptive reaction (e.g. a phobia or anxiety state) may become self-perpetuating even when the original stress is no longer operating. It is then necessary to break the vicious circle by, for example, *behaviour therapy*.

It will already be obvious that what the psychiatrist calls 'psychotherapy' is not altogether different from some activities which are called 'casework' by social workers, or 'counselling' by others. Psychiatrists have no monopoly in the treatment of neuroses and indeed many of them are not very good at it. It is often suggested the so-called 'medical model' ought not to be applied to the neuroses, as it encourages people to feel ill and helpless and discourages them from helping themselves.

The distinction between psychoses and neuroses is fairly crucial since it affects the way a patient is treated, not only by psychiatrists but by other professionals, and the law, and the world in general. *Psychotic* patients are regarded as 'ill' (or 'mad'). Psychotic experiences are outside the normal range and have no parallel in the experience of ordinary people. Psychotic patients often fail to recognize that they are ill. Society does not hold them fully responsible for the results of their actions, and feels justified in making decisions for them, including if necessary compulsory admission to hospital and treatment without consent. Diagnosis is based in part on the presence of various characteristic features. The causes are not wholly 'psychological': stress may be a trigger factor but there are other factors involved that seem to be 'biological', including some which are perhaps genetic. Treatment is on 'medical' lines, including drugs.

Neurotic patients, on the other hand, may be seen as 'ill' but are not usually regarded as 'mad'. Their experiences and behaviour are not entirely different from those of other people, and may strike the observer as an extreme or exaggerated variety of normal experiences, which perhaps the observer has encountered in his own life. This makes them more 'understandable', and it also encourages moral judgements — since the observer may feel that he himself has coped with similar experiences by 'strength of character' or 'self-discipline'. Judgement may be affected in the neuroses, but neurotic patients are likely to be held legally responsible for the consequences of their actions, and they are generally expected to make their own decisions, including decisions about treatment. Neuroses are (roughly speaking) stress reactions. Diagnosis includes understanding the stresses and their underlying psychological causes. Genetic factors are not considered very important. Treatment should include some form of psychotherapy. Drugs merely relieve symptoms.

Comparing these two descriptions, it seems that the distinction depends on two very untidy sets of separate variables, phenomenological, aetiological, and even judgemental. They seem to include:

	Psychosis	*Neurosis*
Comprehensibility:	alien or bizarre	familiar, even if exaggerated.
Supposed causes:	partly 'biological'	'psychological'
Self control:	not possible	possible with effort
Moral attitude:	can't help it	ought to control it

| *Compulsion:* | treatment may be imposed | treatment may not be imposed |
| *If criminal offence is committed:* | treat | punish |

In practice these disparate elements usually hang together well enough to be utilized without too much Procrustean manoeuvering *as long as we stay in one culture*: but when we move across cultures they can easily fall apart. One of the commonest errors is to diagnose a psychosis (usually schizophrenia) because of the incomprehensibility factor, and apply a 'biological' approach when a 'psychological' one would be more appropriate (for examples see chapters 11, 12, and 14). This trap can be avoided by asking, not 'psychotic or neurotic?', but to what extent, or in what ways psychotic or neurotic? In practice psychiatrists usually operate with some flexibility.

Appendix 2
A Guide to Asian Names

(Extract from *Explanation of Asian Names* produced for Bradford Community Relations Council by Rev. Peter Hawkins.)

MUSLIM NAMES

There is a family name (like a surname) from the father's side, e.g. *Rashid*. The son of the family will have a name personal to himself, e.g. *Abdul*. Because he is a Muslim his personal name will be followed or preceded by the title name, e.g. *Mohammed*. His full name is therefore Mohammed Abdul Rashid, and he is addressed verbally as Abdul or Mr Rashid. A daughter of this family will have a personal name, e.g. *Safia*. She will not usually use the family name (*Rashid*), but she will use a title, e.g. *Begum*, *Bibi*, or *Sultana*, following her personal name. Her full name is (e.g.) Safia Begum, and she is addressed as Safia. When she marries she *may* take her husband's family name and become (e.g.) *Safia Lateef Begum*; but she may not take his name, or may prefer not to speak it, in which case her title comes first and she is *Begum Safia*.

SIKH NAMES

There is a family name (like a surname) from the father's side, e.g. *Chahal*. Originally this indicated the Hindu sub-caste from which the family came, and its use was discouraged by the founder of Sikhism, who sought to emphasize the equality of all Sikhs by giving a new family name which is *Singh* (lion) for all Sikh men and *Kaur* (princess) for all Sikh women. However, the commonality of these names (Singh and Kaur) means that they have become titles, and are placed at the middle or end of the name. There is also a personal name (e.g. *Balwant* or *Peramjit*). Sikh personal names do not indicate the sex of the bearer: Balwant or Peramjit can be both a boy's and a girl's name. Sex is indicated by the title; thus the son and daughter of the Chahal house-hold are respectively *Balwant Singh Chahal* and *Peramjit Kaur Chahal*. He may be addressed as Mr Chahal or informally as Balwant (not Mr Balwant). She is addressed as Miss Chahal, or informally as Peramjit (not Miss Peramjit). Because of Sikh disapproval of the sub-caste derivation of family names (see above), Balwant Singh Chahal will often call himself Balwant Singh, and Peramjit Kaur Chahal call herself Peramjit Kaur. They will produce the name Chahal only when questioned. Chahal may not appear on documents at all. If the family name is not in use, the appropriate mode of address is Mr Singh or Miss Kaur. When Peramjit Kaur Chahal marries Sadhu Singh Dhillon she becomes Peramjit Kaur Dhillon and is addressed informally as Peramjit (not Mrs Peramjit) or formally as Mrs Dhillon, or, if the family name is not in use, as Mrs Kaur. It is not correct to address any Sikh women as Miss/Mrs Singh.

HINDU NAMES

There is considerable regional variation: The following rules apply in particular to Gujeratis. There is no family name as such, but the sub-caste name (e.g. *Patel* or *Mistry*) is used as a surname. Usually there are three names, e.g. a man may be called *Ratilal Mangalbhai Patel*. His personal name (by which he is addressed informally) is Ratilal. Formally, he is Mr Patel. His middle name, Mangalbhai, is derived from his father's personal name, Mangal. A single woman may be called, e.g. *Bharatiben Shonabhai Mistry*. Her personal name is Bharatiben and she is addressed by this, or as Bharati (the suffix 'ben' denotes gender). Formally, she is Miss Mistry. Her middle name Shonabhai is derived from her father's personal name, Shona. If Bharatiben Shonabhai Mistry marries Ratilal Mangalbhai Patel, she changes her name to Bharatiben Ratilalbhai Patel, taking her husband's name with the suffix 'bhai' as her new middle name. Their son may be named Jyoti Ratilalbhai Patel, and their daughter Savitaben Ratilalbhai Patel (known as Savita). To complicate matters further, children are often given pet names (e.g. *Kalo*, *Koukou*) which are used within the family until outgrown.

Since all Asian names written in English are transliterations they are phonetic approximations. e.g. a particular Bengali name may be rendered as either Bibekaanondo or Vivekananda, the correct pronounciation being somewhere between the two. Sadique may be written as Siddique, Sadiq, Sidik or Sadik, and it is not possible to say that one spelling is more 'correct' than another.

For further information see *Explanation of Asian Names* (Bradford CRC) or Henley (1979).

Appendix 3
Some Organic Disorders which May Present with Psychiatric Symptoms

Alarmist stories about leprosy and other exotic importations can be largely discounted. For further details see Nnochiri (1970). There are, however, a few conditions which, while not limited to any ethnic group, have a higher incidence among immigrants than among the indigenous population and can present with symptoms which may be misdiagnosed as psychogenic or functional.

Anaemia should always be considered in patients complaining of tiredness, and may be concealed by skin pigmentation. It may be dietary, or due to intestinal infestation, or menorrhagia which the patient is too shy to mention, as well as more obvious causes.

Vitamin D deficiency is common in Asian women, and can present with vague, diffuse pains in bones and joints occurring before there is any clear radiographic evidence of osteomalacia. Absence of physical signs and radiographic confirmation should not prevent a clinical trial or Calcium + Vitamin D tablets in suspected cases.

Tuberculosis, both pulmonary and extrapulmonary, are commoner in non-European countries than in Britain, and the symptoms may be misdiagnosed as functional *either* in the initial stages of tuberculous meningitis *or* due to lassitude and general debility for which there is no obvious cause.

Deafness in different degrees appears to be slightly more prevalent among Asians, and can cause incorrect diagnosis of mental handicap or behaviour disorders in children.

Heavy metal poisoning due to surma or the use of traditional remedies is a possibility which should be kept in mind (see Chapter 19).

Drug interactions: interaction between Karela (a common ingredient of curry, also used medicinally) and Chlorpropamide has been reported (Aslam *et al*. 1979). There may be others, and some of the constituents of medicines prescribed by Hakims have known bioactivity (see Chapter 19).

Epilepsy occurs in all ethnic groups. Its comparative prevalence has not been surveyed, but the less florid manifestations of temporal lobe discharges without Grand Mal, which can present diagnostic problems in any case, are particularly easy to overlook if there are problems of language.

Sexually transmitted diseases usually have increased prevalence in any group of young men who are living apart from their families.

Appendix 4
The Transcultural Psychiatry Unit, Lynfield Mount Hospital, Bradford, Yorkshire

Bradford is an industrial city in the north of England. Historically it was the centre of the wool textile industry which developed in the nineteenth century, conferring great prosperity, but is currently in recession. Because its industries were labour-intensive, Bradford has a long history of immigration, and its population of half a million currently includes about 60,000 who were born outside Britain. The largest single group are from the northern parts of Pakistan and Azad Kashmir, but there are also substantial numbers of Sikhs, Bangla Deshis, Gujeratis, Poles, and West Indians, and smaller numbers from other European countries, Latin America, and Vietnam.

Psychiatric services for the urban centre of Bradford are provided at Lynfield Mount Hospital, which is a 200-bedded unit opened in 1967 adjacent to Bradford Royal Infirmary. It serves a population of 200,000, of whom about 20 per cent are immigrants or their first-generation descendants. In the early 1970s it became apparent to the hospital staff that the mental health provision that they were making for these ethnic minorities was unsatisfactory, mainly because of language difficulties and lack of cultural understanding. To remedy this, a multidisciplinary team of hospital staff came together with the present author as convenor, and it was agreed that all patients referred to the hospital should be treated by this team if linguistic, cultural, or adaptational problems seemed to be significant factors. The first task of the team was to educate itself: this process started with a series of seminars at which members of ethnic minorities came to the hospital to tell the staff about the problems which they and their compatriots were facing and to give instruction on cultural norms, customs, and values, in relation to mental illness and treatment. Self-education and education of others (in and outside the hospital) have remained an important function of the team.

A register is kept of all patients who were born outside Britain or had one or both parents born outside Britain (overinclusive criteria, deliberately). In the period 1974 to 1981 this register has accumulated just over 1,000 names. The majority of these patients have been treated as out-patients; the number of in-patients at any one time varying between two and fifteen, with an average length of stay of about one month, which is not significantly different from indigenous patients. The ratio of compulsory to informal admissions does not differ from indigenous patients.

The constitution of the team has altered over the years. Its current membership (April 1981) is:

PR   Consultant Psychiatrist
JB   Consultant Psychiatrist (speaks Urdu, Punjabi, Pushtu)
SK   Clinical Assistant (GP) (speaks Bengali, Hindi) ⎱ each employed
MS   Clinical Assistant (speaks Punjabi, Urdu) ⎰ 7 hours/week
SHO/Reg/S.Reg Psychiatric trainees in rotation
NF   Social Worker (specialist mental health caseworker, local authority)
WJ   Social Worker (speaks Polish)
AT   Social Work Assistant (speaks Urdu, Bengali, Hindi)
Ward Sister/Charge Nurse(s)
PH   Assistant Anglican Chaplain (speaks Bengali, Hindi, Urdu, Punjabi)
AG   Clinical Psychologist (speaks Hungarian)
PL   Research Assistant

With the exception of AT and PL, all the above have other duties which occupy the majority of their time. The team is very much a part-time team, and while there is at least one member available every day, there is only one day on which they all assemble, which is Wednesday. Wednesdays start with a meeting at 9.00 a.m. on the ward (nearly all 'transcultural' in-patients are on the same ward) during which all patients are reviewed and discussed. After this some of the team have out-patient clinics and others may have individual interviews with in-patients or relatives. There is also a social/therapy group for Polish patients at this time. The team reassembles for a working lunch at which clinical decisions are made on a multidisciplinary basis. In the afternoon the Consultants and Clinical Assistants run four concurrent out-patient clinics, seeing new and follow-up patients individually or together, with social work expertise available as required. By this arrangement it is usually possible for a patient and his or her relatives to talk to at least one person in their own language, and for treatment decisions to incorporate all the necessary information and the contributions of different disciplines.

The Unit's primary responsibility is to patients living within the hospital catchment area, but a flexible policy is adopted. There are some immigrant patients who have no language problem and whose illnesses are not significantly related to adaptation or modified by culture, who can be treated as well or better by one of the other clinical teams attached to the hospital. Increasingly, the advice of the unit is being sought on behalf of patients who live outside the catchment area, or in relation to problems which are not strictly 'psychiatric' and for which hospital referral would be inappropriate. Colleagues seeking advice in such cases are usually invited to join the lunch-time staff meeting.

The Unit is fortunate in having the services of staff who span a wide range of cultural as well as personal and professional backgrounds, and the discussions which take place at the weekly staff meetings constitute an on-going exercise in mutual education from which everyone benefits, the indigenous English members probably most of all. These meetings also serve as an introduction to transcultural psychiatry for trainees, students, and visiting practitioners. Once every month the staff meeting is replaced by an open meeting with a speaker. Recent topics have included Islamic beliefs (by a local Imam); resettlement of refugees (by a Vietnamese social worker); reports of mental health projects in rural Pakistan and India; Sikhism (by a leader of the Sikh community); exiles in old age (by a Polish social worker); discussion of the role of interpreters in the health service; and the problems of Muslim teenagers. These meetings usually attract an audience of 70–100 people including doctors in community health, paediatrics and other specialities, community nurses, health visitors, social workers, teachers, university staff, students in various disciplines, health education specialists and police officers. This seems to indicate a fairly widespread desire for knowledge. Ethnic minority members are usually about 15–20 per cent of the audience and they always take a leading part in discussion.

Although the unit is not primarily geared to research, its members have undertaken some specific projects, and its resources have been used a good deal by other researchers.

The cost of the unit has been very small, since most members of the team were already employed by either the NHS or Local Authority, and contributed part of their time with the approval of their colleagues or departments. The only additional staff are the two visiting Asian doctors who are each paid for two Clinical Assistant sessions per week, and one full-time Social Work Assistant. The Health Authority also contributes by the provision of office accommodation, library facilities, expenses connected with meetings (including a bread-and-cheese lunch), and secretarial time. Several staff members have received bursaries for study tours abroad and attendance at conferences, and a Research Assistant was funded for three years by the Regional Health Authority. None of these, however, are essential prerequisites for the establishment of a specialist service, and there seems no reason why such teams should not come into existence in other cities with comparable populations. As far as we are aware, this has not yet happened.

NOTE

1 Descriptions of the Unit are given in Schlicht and Carmichael (1976); Knight (1978); and Manning (1979).

Appendix 5
Useful Addresses

British Council, Student Welfare Department, 10 Spring Gardens, London SW1A 2BN.

British Medical Anthropology Society, Hon. Sec. A. Williams, Hughes Hall, Cambridge CB1 2EW.

British Refugee Council, 3–9 Bondway, London SW8 1SJ.

Centre for Ethnic Minorities Health Studies, Field House Postgraduate Centre, Bradford Royal Infirmary, Duckworth Lane, Bradford 9.

Commission for Racial Equality, 10–12 Allington Street, London W1 (and Regional Offices: see telephone directory).

Community Health Group for Ethnic Minorities, 28 Churchfield Road, Acton, London W3 6EB.

Community Relations Councils. In most cities: see telephone directories.

Home Office Immigration Department, 50, Queen Anne's Gate, London SW1H 9AT.

International Association for Cross-Cultural Psychology, Secretary General Dr. Y. H. Poortinga, Dept. of Psychology, Tilburg University, 5000 LE Tilburg, Netherlands.

International Social Services, Cranmer House, 39 Brixton Road, London SW9 6DD.

Joint Council for the Welfare of Immigrants, 44 Theobalds Road, London WC1X 8SP.

Kings Fund: The King Edward's Hospital Fund for London, 126 Albert Street, London NW1 7NX.

Mind (National Association for Mental Health), 22, Harley Street, London W1N 2ED.

Minority Rights Group, 36 Craven Street, London WC2N 5NG.

National Association for Asian Youth, 46, High Street, Southall, Middx. UB1 3DB.

Ockenden Venture, Ockenden, Guildford Road, Woking, Surrey, GU22 7UU.

Refugee Action, 36 Bayswater Row, Leeds 6.

Runnymede Trust, Victoria Chambers, 16–18 Strutton Ground, London SW1P 2HP.

Transcultural Psychiatry Society (UK), Hon. Sec. Dr. J. Cox, University Dept. of Psychiatry, Royal Edinburgh Hospital, Morningside, Edinburgh EH10 5HF.

Transcultural Psychiatry Unit, Lynfield Mount Hospital, Heights Lane, Bradford BD9 6DP.

United Kingdom Immigrants Advisory Service, Brettenham House, 7th Floor, Savoy Street, Strand, London WC2E 7EP (and regional offices: see telephone directories).

Appendix 6
Treatment of Overseas Visitors under the NHS

For details see National Health Service (Charges for Overseas Visitors) Regulations 1982. All persons who are legally resident in Britain and all visitors who have been in Britain more than one year are entitled to free treatment. In addition, free treatment is available to nationals of the following countries with which Britain has reciprocal arrangements: Austria, Bulgaria, Czechoslovakia, Denmark, West Germany, East Germany, Hong Kong, Hungary, New Zealand, Norway, Poland, Portugal, Rumania, Sweden, Yugoslavia, Channel Islands, Gibraltar, Isle of Man, Malta, and USSR and to all nationals of EEC countries. The following are also exempt from charges: people coming to Britain to work; wives, and children under 18, of people settled in Britain; British residents who work abroad (under certain conditions); refugees; seamen in UK registered vessels; and offshore workers.

There is no charge for emergency treatment in Accident and Emergency Out-Patient Departments, nor to treatment of communicable diseases. Psychiatric patients are exempt from charges if compulsorily detained in hospital, but not otherwise. The regulations are mandatory. Health Authorities have been instructed what scales of charges to use, and how to decide eligibility. The regulations are operational from October 1982. Many who have studied them, including the present author, consider them regrettable and foresee great problems in implementation (see p. 205).

References

Aceves, J. (1971) *Social Change in a Spanish Village*. Cambridge, Mass.: Schenkman.

Ackernacht, E. H. (1948) (quoted in Rao, A. V. (1966)). Depression — A Psychiatric Analysis of Thirty Cases. *Indian Journal of Psychiatry* 8(2): 143-54.

Adomakoh, C. (1975) The Pattern of Depressive Illness in Africans. In T. Asuni (ed.) (1975) *Recognition of Depression in the African.* (Proceedings of round table discussion 3 July 1975, IV Pan-African Congress on Psychiatry). Sarl, Abidjan: Ciba-Geigy.

Adorno, T. W., Frenkel-Brunswick, E., Levinson, D. J. and Sandford, R. N. (1950) *The Authoritarian Personality*. New York: Harper.

Ahmed, H. (1977) Culture's Influence on Delusions. *Psychiatrica Clinicia* 11(1): 1-9.

Ahmed, S. (1978) Asian Girls and Culture Conflict. *Social Work Today* 9(47): 14-16. Reprinted in Cheetham *et al.* (eds) *Social and Community Work in a Multi-Racial Society.* London: Open University Press/Harper & Row 1981.

Ali, A. R., Smales, O. R. C., and Aslam, M. (1978) Surma and Lead Poisoning. *British Medical Journal* 30 September: 915-16.

Allen, J. J., Rack, P. H., and Vaddadi, K. S. (1977) Differences in the Effects of Clomipramine on English and Asian Volunteers: Preliminary Report on a Pilot Study. *Postgraduate Medical Journal* 53 Supplement 4.79.

Ambelas, A. (1979) Psychologically Stressful Events in the Precipitation of Manic Episodes. *British Journal of Psychiatry* 135(15).

Anon (1981) Babylon System. In *Finding Me* (Anthology). Sheffield: Hub Publications.

Anwar, M. (1979) *The Myth of Return.* London: Heinemann.

Anwar, M. and Little, A. (1976) *Between Two Cultures: A Study of Relationships between Generations in the Asian Community in Britain.* London: Commission for Racial Equality.

Aslam, M. (1979) 'The Practice of Asian Medicine in the United Kingdom'. Thesis for Ph.D., Dept. of Pharmacy, University of Nottingham (unpublished).

Aslam, M. and Davis, S. S. (1979a) The Hakim and His Role in the Immigrant Community: Report to the Department of Health and Social Security 1979. Unpublished.

———— (1979b) The Practice of Asian Medicine in the United Kingdom and the Role of the Visiting Hakim. *Medicos* 4(2).

Aslam, M., Davis, S. S., and Fletcher, R. F. (1979) Compliance in Medication by Asian Immigrants. *Nursing Times* 75(22): 931.

Aslam, M., Davis, S. S. and Healy, M. A. (1979) Heavy Metals in Some Asian Medicines and Cosmetics. *Public Health* 93: 274–84.

Aslam, M., Davis, S. S., Farrar, N., and Rack, P. H. (in press) *Health Care needs of Asians in the U. K.* 3rd International Congress on Rehabilitation, Orebro, Sweden, September 1978.

Aslam, M., Healy, M. A., Davis, S. S., and Ali, A. R. (1980) *Surma and Blood Lead in Children. Lancet* 1: 658–59.

Aslam, M. and Stockley, I. H. (1979) Interaction Between Curry Ingredient (Karela) and Drug (Chlorpropamide). *Lancet* 1: 607.

Astrup, C. and Ødegaard, O. (1960). Internal Migration and Mental Disease in Norway. *Psychiatric Quarterly,* Supplement 34: 116.

Babcock, J. W. (1954) Cited in Hoch and Zubin (eds) *Depression.* New York: Orme and Stratton.

Bagley, C. (1968) Migration, Race and Mental Health: A Review of Some Recent Literature. *Race* IX: 343.

———— (1969) A Survey of Problems Reported by Indian and Pakistani Immigrants in Britain. *Race* IX: 65.

———— (1971a) Mental Illness in Immigrant Minorities in London. *Journal of Biosocial Science* 3: 449–59.

———— (1971b) The Social Aetiology of Schizophrenia in Immigrant Groups. *International Journal of Social Psychiatry* 17: 292–304.

———— (1972) A Comparative Study of Mental Illness among Immigrant Groups in Britain. *Ethnics* 1: 23–36.

———— (1975) Sequels of Alienation: A Social Psychological View of the Adaptation of West Indian Migrants in Britain. In Glaser (ed.) *Case Studies in Human Rights and Fundamental Freedoms.* Vol. 2. The Hague: NIJHOFF.

———— (1976) *Behavioural Deviance in Ethnic Minority Children. A Review of Published Studies.* London: New Community.

Bagley, C. and Binitie, A. (1970) Alcoholism and Schizophrenia in Irishmen in London. *British Journal of Addiction* 65: 3–7.

Bailey, F. G. (1966) The Peasant View of the Bad Life. Reprinted in

T. Shanin (ed.) *Peasants and Peasant Societies* (1971). Harmondsworth: Penguin.

Bal, Pash (1981) Communicating with Non-English-Speaking Patients. *British Medical Journal* **283**: 368.

Ballard, C. (1979) Conflict, Continuity and Change: Second Generation South Asians. In Saifullah Khan (ed.) *Minority Families in Britain: Support and Stress*. London: Macmillan.

Ballard, R. (1977) The Sikhs: The Development of South Asian Settlements in Britain. In J. L. Watson (ed.) *Between Two Cultures* Oxford: Blackwell.

——— (1979) Ethnic Minorities and the Social Services. In V. Saifullah Khan (ed.) *Minority Families in Britain: Support and Stress*. London: Macmillan.

Batta, I. D., McCulloch, J. W., and Smith, N. J. (1965) A Study of Juvenile Delinquency among Asians and Half-Asians. *British Journal of Criminology* **15**(1): 32–42.

Batta, I. D. Mawby, R. I., and McCulloch, J. W. (1980) *Children in Local Authority Care: A Monitoring of Racial Differences in Bradford.* (In press.)

Bavington, J. (1981) Depression in Pakistan. Transcultural Psychiatry Society (UK) Workshop, Leeds, April. (Unpublished.)

Berger, J. and Mohr, J. (1967) *A Fortunate Man: The Story of a Country Doctor.* Harmondsworth: Penguin.

——— (1975) *Seventh Man.* Harmondsworth: Penguin.

Bhatti, F. M. (1976) Language Difficulties and Social Isolation: The Case of South Asian Women in Britain. *New Community* **115**.

Binder, R. L. and Levy, R. (1981) Extrapyramidal Reactions in Asians. *American Journal of Psychiatry* **138**(9): 1243–244.

Binitie, A. (1975) The Differentiation of Masked Depression from Psychoneurotic Disorders. In T. Asuni (ed.) Recognition of Depression on the African. (Proceedings of a Round Table Discussion, 3 July 1975, IV Pan-African Congress on Psychiatry.) Sarl, Abidjan: Ciba-Geigy.

Boatswain, Hugh (1981) Old Father (Poem) In J. Berry (ed.) *Bluefoot Traveller: Poetry by West Indians in Britain.* London: Harrap.

Boaz, F. (1940) *Race, Language and Culture.* 1966 editon. New York: The Free Press.

Bordieu, P. (1963) The Attitude of the Algerian Peasant Towards Time. In J. Pitt-Rivers (ed.) *Mediterranean Countrymen.* The Hague: Mouton Co.

Bottoms, A. (1973) Crime and Delinquency in Immigrant and Minority Groups. In P. Watson (ed.) *Psychology and Race.* Harmondsworth: Penguin.

Bradford, City of, Metropolitan Council (1982) *Policy Statement on Race Relations*. Bradford: City Hall.

Bram, G. (1979) The Psychological Problems of Elderly Refugees. Paper presented at Seminar of Elderly Refugees, 27 June 1979; London. British Red Cross Society, 9 Grosvenor Crescent.

Branch, R. A., Salih, S. Y., and Homoda, M. (1978) Racial Differences in Drug Metabolizing Activity: Study with Antipyrine in the Sudan. *Clinical Pharmacology and Therapy* **24**: 283.

Brandon, D. (1979) The Prevalence of Psychiatric Problems among Ethnic Minorities in England and Wales. London: MIND (unpublished).

Brown, R. (1965) *Social Psychology*. London: Collier-Macmillan.

Burke, A. W. (1973) The Consequences of Unplanned Repatriation. *British Journal of Psychiatry* **123**(527): 109.

Carothers, J. C. (1947) A Study of Mental Derangement in Africans. *Journal of Mental Science* **93**. 548–97.

———— (1951) Frontal Lobe Function and the African. *Journal of Mental Science* **97**: 12.

———— (1953) *The African Mind in Health and Disease*. Geneva: W H O.

Carpenter, L. and Brockington, I. F. (1980) A Study of Mental Illness in Asians, West Indians and Africans living in Manchester. *British Journal of Psychiatry* **137**: 201.

Carstairs, G. M. (1956) Hinjra and Jiryan. *British Journal of Medical Psychology* **29**: 128.

———— (1958a) *The Twice Born: A Study of a Community of High-Caste Hindus*. Bloomington: Indiana University Press.

———— (1958b) Some Problems of Psychiatry in Patients from Alien Cultures. *Lancet*: 1217–20.

———— (1975) Measuring Psychiatric Morbidity in a South Indian Population. *Bulletin of the British Psychological Society* **28**: 95–101.

Carstairs, G. M. and Kapur, R. L. (1976) *The Great Universe of Kota: Stress, Change, and Mental Disorder in an Indian Village*. London: Hogarth Press.

Castles, S. and Kusack, G. (1973) *Immigrant Workers and Class Structure in Western Europe*. Oxford: Oxford University Press.

Chandrasena, R. (1979) Phenomenology of Mental Disorder among the West Indian and West African-born Patients in Hackney. Transcultural Psychiatry Society Workshop, London, November 1979. (Unpublished.)

Chowdhury, A. K. M. N. (1966) Admission to an East Pakistan Mental Hospital. *British Journal of Psychiatry* **112**: 65–8.

CIMADE (Comité Inter-Mouvement Auprès des Evacués) (1981) The Influence of Political Repression and Exile on Children. In *Mental*

Health and Latin-American Exiles. London: World University Serivce.

Clare, A. E. (1974) Mental Illness in the Irish Emigrant. *Journal of the Irish Medical Association* 67: 20.

Clarke, E. (1979) Imagery of Madness. Transcultural Psychiatry Workshop, London, November 1979. (Unpublished.)

Clark, K. B. and Clark, M. P. (1939) The Development of Consciousness of Self and the Emergence of Racial Identification in Negro Pre-School Children. *Journal of Social Psychology* 10: 591–99.

Cochrane, R. (1977) Mental Illness in Immigrants to England and Wales: An Analysis of Mental Hospital Admissions 1971. *Social Psychiatry* 12: 25.

—— (1979) Psychological and behavioural disturbance in West Indians and Pakistanis in Britain. *British Journal of Psychiatry* 134: 201–10.

—— (1980) A Comparative Evaluation of the Symptom Rating Test and the Langner 22-Item Index for Use in Epidemiological Surveys. *Psychological Medicine* 10: 115–24.

Cochrane, R., Hashmi, F., and Stopes-Roe, M. (1977) Measuring Psychological Disturbance in Asian Immigrants to Britain. *Social Science and Medicine* II: 157–64.

Cochrane, R. and Stopes-Roe, M. (1977) Psychological and Social Adjustment of Asian Immigrants to Britain: A Community Survey. *Social Psychology* 12: 195.

—— (1981) Psychological Symptom Levels in Indian Immigrants to England: A Comparison with Native English. *Psychological Medicine* 11: 319–27.

COLAT (The Latin American Social Work Collective) (1981) Towards a Libertarian Therapy for Latin American Exiles. In *Mental Health and Exile: Papers Arising from a Seminar on Mental Health and Latin American Exiles.* London: World University Service.

Community Relations Commission (1977) *Urban Deprivation, Racial Inequality and Social Policy: A Report.* London: HMSO.

Constantinides, P. (1977) The Greek Cypriots: Factors in the Maintenance of Ethnic Identity. In J. L. Watson (ed.) *Between Two Cultures.* Oxford: Blackwell.

Coombe, V. (1976) Health and Social Services and Minority Ethnic Groups. *Royal Society of Health Journal* 96(1): 34. (Cited by Storer.)

Copeland, J. R. M. (1968) Aspects of Mental Illness in West African Students. *International Journal of Social Psychiatry* 3: 7–13.

Cox, J. (1976) Psychiatric Assessment and the Immigrant Patient. *British Journal of Hospital Medicine* 16: 38–40.

Cross, C. (1978) *Ethnic Minorities in the Inner City: The Ethnic*

Dimension in Urban Deprivation in England. London: Commission for Racial Equality.

Curle, A. (1971) *Making Peace.* London: Tavistock.

Dahya, B. (1973) Pakistanis in Britain: Transients or Settlers? *Race* **XIV**(3): 241–77.

Danna, J. J. (1980) Migration and Mental Illness: What Role do Traditional Childhood Socialization Practices Play? *Cultural Medicine and Psychiatry* **4**: 25–42.

Dastur, J. F. (1960) *Everybody's Guide to Agurvedic Medicine.* Bombay: Taraporevala Ltd.

Davidson, S. (1979a) Long-Term Psychosocial Sequelae in Holocaust Survivors and their Families. *Israel-Netherlands Symposium on The Impact of Persecution, Jerusalem, 1977.* Rijswijk, Netherlands: Ministry of Cultural Affairs.

—— (1979b) Massive Trauma and Social Support. *Journal of Psychosomatic Support* **23**: 395–402.

—— (1980a) The Clinical Effects of massive Psychic Trauma in Families of Holocaust Survivors. *Journal of Marital and Family Therapy* **6**: 11–21.

—— (1980b) Transgenerational Transmission in the Families of Holocaust Survivors. *International Journal of Family Psychiatry* **1**: 95–113.

Davis, S. S. and Aslam, M. (1979) Eastern Treatment for Eastern Health? *Journal of Community Nursing* May 1979: 16–20. Reprinted in Cheetham *et al.* (1981) *Social and Community Work in a Multi-Racial Society.* London: Harper and Row/Open University Press.

Dean, G., Walsh, D., Downing, H., and Shelley, E. (1981) First Admissions of Native Born and Immigrants to Psychiatric Hospitals in South-East England 1976. *British Journal of Psychiatry* **139**: 506–12.

Denber, H. C. B. and Bente, D. (1967) Clinical Response to Pharmacotherapy in Different Settings. In *Neuropsychopharmacology* (H. Brill *et al.* (eds): 517. New York Excerpta Medica Foundation ICS 129.

Denber, H. C. B. and Collard, J. (1962) Différences de Bioreactivité au Haloperiodot entre Deux Groupes de Psychotiques, Americain et Européen. *Acta Neurologica et Psychiatrica Belgica* **62**: 577.

Denber, H. C. B., Bente, D., and Rajotte, P. (1962) Comparative Analysis of the Action of Butyrylperazine in Manhattan State Hospital and the University Psychiatric Clinic at Erlangen. *American Journal of Psychiatry* **119**: 203.

Devereux, G. (1956) Normal and Abnormal Reprinted 1980 in *Basic Problems of Ethnopsychiatry.* Translated by Gulati and Devereux. American Edition. Chicago: University of Chicago Press.

Dharamsi, F. H. (1976) Ethnic Minorities and Mental Health. Institute of Social Welfare Seminar, University of Nottingham, March 1976 (unpublished).

Dobrowolski, K. (1971) Peasant Traditional Culture. In T. Shanin, (ed.) *Peasants and Peasant Societies*. Harmondsworth: Penguin.

Driver, G. (1979) Classroom and School Achievement: West Indian Adolescents and Their Teachers. In V. Saifullah Khan (ed.) *Minority Families in Britain: Support and Stress*. London: Macmillan.

D'Souza, F. (1980) *The Refugee Dilemma*. London: Minority Rights Group.

Eaton, W. W. and Lasry, J. C. (1978) Mental Health and Occupational Mobility in a Group of Immigrants. *Social Science and Medicine* 12: 53–8.

Eitinger, L. (1959) The Incidence of Mental Disease among Refugees in Norway. *Journal of Mental Science* 105: 326–380.

—— (1960) The Symptomatology of Mental Illness among Refugees in Norway. *Journal of Mental Science* 106: 947.

—— (1981) Foreigners in our time: Historical survey on psychiatry's approach to migration and refugee status. In Eitinger L. and Schwarz D. (eds.) *Strangers in the World*. Bern: Hans Huber.

Eitinger, L. and Grünfeld, B. (1966) Psychoses among Refugees in Norway *Acta Psychiatrica Scandinavia* 42: 315–28.

Eitinger, L. and Schwarz, D. (eds) (1981) *Strangers in the World*. Bern: Hans Huber.

Eysenck, H. J. (1971) *Race, Intelligence and Education*. London: Temple Smith.

Faergeman, P. M. (1963) *Psychogenic Psychoses*. London: Butterworths.

Fanon, F. (1961) *The Wretched of the Earth*. English Edition 1967. Harmondsworth: Penguin.

Farrar, N. (1981) Working with Immigrants in a Psychiatric Setting. Bradford Social Services Directorate (unpublished).

Fernando, N. P., Heacy, M. A., Aslam, M., Davis, S. S., and Hussain, A., (1981) Lead Poisoning and Traditional Practices: The Consequences for World Health. *Public Health* 95: 250–60.

Fernando, S. J. M. (1966) Depressive Illness in Jews and Non-Jews. *British Journal of Psychiatry* 112: 491.

—— (1969) Cultural Differences in the Hostility of Depressed Patients. *British Journal of Medical Psychology* 42: 67.

—— (1975) A Cross-Cultural Study of some Familial and Social Factors in Depressive Illness. *British Journal of Psychiatry* 127.

Ferron, O. (1973) Family, Marital and Childrearing Patterns in Different Ethnic Groups. In P. Watson (ed.) *Psychology and Race*. Harmondsworth: Penguin.

Foner, N. (1977) The Jamaicans: Cultural and Social Change among

Migrants in Britain. In J. L. Watson (ed.) *Between Two Cultures*. Oxford: Blackwell.

Foster, G. M. (1965) *Tzintzuntzan: Mexican Peasants in a Changing World*. Boston: Little, Brown.

—— (1967) Peasant Society and the Image of Limited Good. *American Anthropologist* **67**: 2. Reprinted in J. M. Potter, M. N. Diaz, and G. M. Foster (eds) *Peasant Society: A Reader*. Boston: Little, Brown.

—— (1973) *Traditional Societies and Technological Change*. New York/London: Harper and Row.

Fowler, N. (Secretary of State for Social Services) (1982) in DHSS Press Release 82/46 'Most Overseas Visitors to Pay Full Cost of Hospital Treatment'. London: DHSS 22.2.82.

Franklin, J. H. (1966) A Brief History of the Negro in the United States. In J. P. Davis (ed.) *The American Negro Reference Book*. Englewood Cliffs: Prentice-Hall.

Fraser, M. S., Bulpitt, C. J., Khan, C., Mould, G., Mucklow, J. C., and Dolliery, C. T. (1976) Factors Affecting Antipyrine Metabolism in West African Villagers. *Clinical Pharmacology and Therapeutics* **20**: 369.

Freud, S. (1917) *Mourning and Melancholia*. Standard Edition (1957) Vol. 14: 243-58. London: Hogarth Press.

Friedman, F. G. (1953) The World of La Miseria. *Partisan Review* **20**: 218-31.

Frost, I. (1938) Home-sickness and Immigrant Psychoses. *Journal of Mental Science* **84**: 801-47.

Gallaher, J. and Copeland, J. (1972) Compulsory Psychiatric Admission by the Police. *Medicine, Science, and the Law.*

Giggs, J. (1973) High Rates of Schizophrenia Among Immigrants to Nottingham. *Nursing Times* **69**: 1210-212.

Goody, E. N. and Groothves, C. M. (1977) The West Africans: The Quest for Education. In J. L. Watson (ed.) *Between Two Cultures*. Oxford: Blackwell.

Gordon, E. B. (1965) Mentally Ill West Indian Immigrants *British Journal of Psychiatry* **111**: 877-87.

Green, S. D. R., Lealman, G. T. Aslam, M., and Davis, S. S. (1979) Surma and Blood Concentrations. *Public Health* **93**: 371-76.

Haley, A. (1977) *Roots*. London: Pan Books.

Harris, S. (1973) Spearhead of British Racialism. *Patterns of Prejudice* **7**(4): 15-19.

Hashmi, F. (1966) Moves, Migration and Mental Illness. In CIBA Foundation Report: *Immigration, Medical and Social Aspects.*

—— (1968) Community Psychiatric Problems among Birmingham

Immigrants. *British Journal of Social Psychiatry* 2(3): 196–201.
—— (1969) *The Pakistani Family in Britain*. London: Commission for Racial Equality.

Hemsi, L. K. (1967) Psychiatric Mordbidity of West Indian Immigrants. *Social Psychiatry* 2(3): 100.

Henley, A. (1979) *The Asian Patient in Hospital and at Home* London: The Kings Fund.

Hill, D. (1975) Personality Factors among Adolescents in Minority Ethnic Groups. *Education Studies* Vol. 1.

Hitch, P. J. (1975) Migration and Mental Illness in a Northern City. Thesis for Ph.D., Bradford University (unpublished).

—— (1977) Culture, Social Structure and Explanation of Migrant Mental Illness *Mental Health and Society* 4(3–4): 136–43.

—— (1981) Immigration and Mental Health: Local Research and Social Explanations. CRE: *New Community* IX(2): 256.

Hitch, P. J. and Clegg, P. (1980) Modes of Referral of Overseas Immigrant and Native Born First Admissions to Psychiatric Hospital. *Social Science and Medicine* 14A: 369–74.

Hitch, P. J. and Rack, P. H. (1980) Mental Illness among Polish and Russian Refugees in Bradford. *British Journal of Psychiatry* 137: 206–11.

Hoggart, R. (1958) *The Uses of Literacy*. Harmondsworth: Penguin.

Hoijer, H. (1974) *Language, Culture and Society*. Cambridge, Mass.: Winthrop.

Hollingshead, A. B. and Redlich, F. C. (1958) *Social Class and Mental Illness: A Community Study*. New York: John Wiley and Sons.

Horne, A. D. (1978) 'A Study of Ante-Natal Care Uptake amongst Asians in Bradford'. Health Education Department, Bradford. (Unpublished: quoted by Rowell and Rack 1979.)

Hussein, M. F. (1976) 'Affective disorders in Asian immigrants'. *International Congress of Transcultural Psychiatry*. Bradford 1976 (unpublished).

Itil, T. M. (1975) Transcultural psychopharmacology from the EEG point of view. In T. M. Itil (ed.) *Transcultural Neuro-psychopharmacolocy*. Istanbul: Bozak Publishing Co.

Jackson, J. A. (ed.) (1969) *Migration: Sociological Studies*. Cambridge: Cambridge University Press.

Jagucki, W. (1981) *Refugees: Forty Years Later*. SCOR Conference, Haslemere, 9.8.1981 (unpublished).

Johnson, S. C. (1966) *A History of Emigration from the United Kingdom to North America*. London: Frank Cass.

Joseph, R. (1978) Admission of Asian patients to Lynfield Mount Hospital, Bradford. Research Project, University of Leeds (unpublished).

Kardiner, A. and Ovesey, L. (1951) *The Mark of Oppression.* New York: W. W. Norton.

Kellecher, M. J. and Copeland, J. R. M. (1972) *Medicine, Science and the Law* July 220–24.

Kendall, R. E. (1972) Schizophrenia: the Remedy for Diagnostic Confusion. *Journal of Hospital Medicine* October 1972: 383–89.

—— (1975) *The Role of Diagnosis in Psychiatry.* Oxford: Blackwell.

Kessel, W. I. N. (1965) Are Internation Comparisons Timely? Reprinted (1968) in R. M. Acheson (ed.) *Comparability in International Epidemiology.* New York: Milbank Memorial Fund.

Kiernan, V. G. (1979) Introduction in C. Holmes (ed.) *Immigrants and Minorities in British Society.* London: Allen and Unwin.

Kiev, A. (1963) Beliefs and delusions of West Indian Immigrants to London. *British Journal of Psychiatry* **109**: 356–63.

—— (1964) Psychiatric Illness among West Indians in London. *Race* **5**: 48.

—— (1965) Psychiatric morbidity of West Indian immigrants in an Urban Group Practice. *British Journal of Psychiatry* **111**: 51–56.

—— (1972) *Transcultural Psychiatry.* New York: The Free Press.

Kino, F. F. (1951) Aliens Paranoid Reaction. *Journal of Mental Science* **97**: 589–94.

—— (1951) Aliens' Paranoid Reaction. *Journal of Mental Science* **97**: 589–94.

Kleinman, A. M. (1977) Depression, Somatisation, and the New Cross-Cultural Psychiatry. *Social Science and Medicine* **11**: 3–10.

Knight, L. (1978) Protect their Minds Too. *Mind Out* **31**: 12.

Kroeber, A. L. (1948) *Anthropology.* New York: Harcourt Brace Jovanovitch.

Krumperman, A. (1981) Psychosocial Problems of Violence, Especially its Effects on Refugees. Paper at seminar on psychosocial problems of refugees, 9th August 1981. Haslemere, London: British Refugee Council.

Krupinski, J., Schaechter, F., and Cade, J. F. J. (1965) Factors Influencing the Incidence of Mental Disorders among Immigrants. *Medical Journal of Australia* **2**: 269.

Krupinski, J. and Stoller, A. (1975) Incidence of Mental Disorders in Victoria According to Country of Birth *Medical Journal of Australia* **2**: 265.

Krupinski J., Stoller, A., and Wallace, L. (1973) Psychiatric Disorders in Eastern European Refugees now in Australia. *Social Science and Medicine* **7**: 31.

Kunz, (1973) The Refugees in Flight: Kinetic Modesl and Forms of Displacement. *International Migration Review* **7**: 125–46.

Ladbury, S. (1977) The Turkish Cypriots: Ethnic Relations in London and Cyprus. In J. L. Watson (ed.) *Between Two Cultures*. Oxford: Blackwell.

Laing, R. D. (1960) *The Divided Self*. London: Tavistock.

—— (1967) *The Politics of Experience and the Bird of Paradise* Harmondsworth: Penguin.

Laing, R. D. and Esterson, A. (1964) *Sanity, Madness and the Family* London: Tavistock.

Leff, J. P. (1973) Culture and the Differential of Emotional States. *British Journal of Psychiatry* **123**: 299–306.

—— (1974) Transcultural Influences on Psychiatrists' Rating of Verbally Expressed Emotion. *British Journal of Psychiatry* **74**(125): 336.

Leff, J. P. (1976), Fischer, M., and Bertebren, A. A Cross-National Epidemological Study of Mania. *British Journal of Psychiatry* **129**: 428–37.

—— (1977) The Cross Cultural Study of Emotions. *Culture, Medicine and Psychiatry* **I**: 317–50.

—— (1981) *Psychiatry Around the Globe: a Transcultural View*. Basel: Marcel Decker.

Leighton, A. H., Lambo, T. A., Hughes, C. C., Leighton, D. C., Murphy, J. M., and Macklin, D. M. (1963) *Psychiatric Disorder among the Yoruba*. Ithaca: Cornell University Press.

Lewis, I. M. (1971) *Ecastatic Religion: An Anthropological Study of Spirit Possession and Shamanism*. Harmondsworth: Penguin.

—— (1976) *Social Anthropology in Perspective*. Harmondsworth: Penguin.

Lewis, O. (1951) *Life in a Mexican Village: Tepoztlan Restudied*. Urbane: University of Illinois Press.

Lewis, P., Vaddadi, K. S., Rack, P. H., and Allen, J. J. (1980) Ethnic Differences in Drug Response. *Postgraduate Medical Journal* **56** Supplement 1: 46–9.

Lipsedge, M. and Littlewood, R. (1979) Recent Advances in Transcultural Psychiatry. In Granville-Grossman (ed.) *Recent Advances in Clinical Psychiatry: III*. London: Churchill Livingstone.

Littlewood, R. and Cross, S. (1980) Ethnic Minorities and Psychiatric Services. *Sociology of Health and Illness*. 2(2): 195–201.

Littlewood, R. and Lipsedge, M. (1977a) Migration, Ethnicity and Diagnosis. *Psychiatric Clinica* **11**: 15.

—— (1977b) Acute Psychotic Reactions in Migrants. *Bulletin of the Royal College of Psychiatrists* November 1977.

—— (1981) Acute Psychotic Reactions in Caribbean-born Patients. *Psychological Medicine* **11**: 303–18.

—— (1982) *Aliens and Alienists*. Harmondsworth: Penguin.

Lowenthal, D. (1972) *West Indian Societies*. London: Oxford University Press/Institute of Race Relations.

Lucas, C. J., Sainsbury, P., and Collins, J. F. (1962) A Social and Clinical Study of Delusions in Schizophrenia. *Journal of Mental Science* **108**: 747.

Maclean, U. (1971) *Magical Medicine: A Nigerian Case Study*. Harmondsworth: Penguin.

Madan, R. (1979) *Coloured Minorities in Britain: A Comprehensive Bibliography 1970-77*. London: Aldwych Press.

Mahy, G. (1976) The Psychotic West Indian Returns from England International Congress of Transcultural Psychiatry, Bradford 1976 (unpublished).

Mahy, G. (1974) The Structure of the West Indian Family. In R. Prince and D. Barrier (eds) *Configurations*. Lexington: D. C. Heath.

Malzberg, B. (1955) *Mental Hygiene* **19**: 635-60.

—— (1969) Are Immigrants Psychologically Disturbed? In S. C. Ploy and R. E. Edgerton (eds) *Changing Perspectives in Mental Illness*. New York: Holt, Rinehart, and Winston.

Manning, M. (1979) Transcultural Psychiatry. *Community Care*, 25.2.79: 19-21.

Marshall, W. K. (1968) Notes on Peasant Development in the West Indies since 1838. *Social and Economic Studies* **17**: 3. Jamaica: UWI Institute of Social and Economic Research.

Mawby, R. I., McCulloch, J. W., and Batta, I. D. (1979) Crime among Asian Juveniles in Bradford. *International Journal of Sociology of Law* **7**: 297-306.

Mazrui, A. (1979) The Reith Lectures 1979. London: BBC Publications.

Memmi, A. (1957) *Portrait du Colonisé Precedé du Portrait de Colonisateur*. Corres: Buchet/Chastel. English translation (translated by H. Greenfield) published as *The Coloniser and the Colonised*. London: Souvenir Press 1974.

Mezey, A. G. (1960a) Personal Background, Emigration and Mental Disorder in Hungarian Refugees. *Journal of Mental Science* **106**:

—— (1960b) Psychiatric Illness in Hungarian Refugees. *Journal of Mental Science* **106**: 628.

—— (1960c) Psychiatric Aspects of Human Migrations. *International Journal of Social Psychiatry* **5**: 245-60.

Milner, P. (1975) *Children and Race*. Harmondsworth: Penguin.

Montague, A. (1975) *Race and I Q*. New York: Oxford University Press.

Montero, D. (1979) Vietnamese Refugees in America: Toward A Theory of Spontaneous International Migration. *International Migration Review* **13**(4): 624-48.

Moore, T. (1977) An Experimental Language Handicap (personal account). *Bulletin of the British Psychological Society* (1977) **30**: 107–10.

Morice, R. (1978) Psychiatric diagnosis in a transcultural setting: the importance of lexical categories. *British Journal of Psychiatry* **132**: 87–95.

Morris, K. L. (1966) *On Afro-West Indian Thinking.* Reprinted in D. Lowenthal and L. Comitas (eds.) (1973) *The Aftermath of Sovereignty: West Indian Perspectives.* New York: Anchor Press/Doubleday.

Morris, R. and Murphy, E. (1975) *Alcohol Offenders: Court and Community.* Helping Hand Organization.

Mubbashar, M. (1976) Cultural Variation in Depressive Symptomatology. Presented at International Congress on Transcultural Psychiatry, University of Bradford. (Unpublished.)

Munoz, L. (1980 Exile as Bereavement: Socio-Psychological Manifestations of Chilean Exiles in Great Britain. *British Journal of Medical Psychology* **53**: 227–32.

Murphy, H. B. M. (1955) Refugee Psychoses in Great Britain: Admissions to Mental Hospitals. In *Flight and Resettlement.* Paris: UNESCO (1965a) Migration and the Major Mental Diseases. In M. B. Kantor (ed.) *Mobility and Mental Health.*

—— (1965b) *The Epidemiological Approach to Transcultural Psychiatric Research.* CIBA Foundation Symposium, London, February 1965.

—— (1969a) Ethnic Variations in Drug Response *Transcultural Psychiatry Research Review* **VI**: 5.

—— (1969b) *Psychiatric Concomitants of Fusion in Plural Societies.* Proceedings of the Conference Social Change and Cultural Factors in Mental Health in Asia and the Pacific. Honolulu, March 1969.

—— (1973) The Low Rate of Mental Hospitalization Shown by Immigrants to Canada. In C. A. Zwingmann and M. Pfeiffer-Amande (eds) *Uprooting and After.* New York: Springer-Verlag.

—— (1973) Migration and the Major Mental Disorders: A Reappraisal. In C. A. Zwingmann and M. Pfeiffer-Amande (eds) *Uprooting and After.* New York: Springer-Verlag.

—— (1977) Migration, Culture and Mental Health. *Psychological Medicine* **7**: 677–84.

—— (1982) *Comparative Psychiatry: The International and Intercultural Distribution of Mental Illness.* New York: Springer-Verlag.

Murphy, H. B. M., Saunier, M., and Vachon-Spilka, I. (1968) *The Comparability of Psychiatric Assessments in Different Languages and Cultures.* Quebec: Federal-Provincial Mental Health Project 604.7.550 Final report.

Murphy, H. B. Wittkower, E. D., and Chance, N. A. (1964)•A Cross-Cultural Inquiry into the Symptomatology of Depression. *Transcultural Psychiatry Research Review.*

Murphy H. B., Wittkower, E. D., and Chance, N. A. (1967) A Cross-Cultural Inquiry into the Symptamtology of Depression. *International Journal of Psychiatry* **3**: 6–15.

McCulloch, J. W., Smith, N. J., and Batta, I. D. (1974) A Comparative Study of Adult Crime amongst Asians and their Host Population. *Professional Views,* August 1974: 37–9.

McCulloch, J. W., Smith, N. J., and Batta, I. D. (1975) A Study of Juvenile Delinquency among Asians and Half-Asians. *British Journal of Criminology,* January.

Neki, J. S. (1973) Psychiatry in South East Asia *British Journal of Psychiatry* **123**: 257–69.

Nguyen, S. A. N. (1980) The Refugee Experience: A Conceptual Model of Social Disintegration. The Homewood Sanatorium, Guelph, Ontario, Canada (unpublished).

Nicolson, C. (1974) *Strangers to England: Immigration to England 1100-1952.* London: Wayland.

Nnochiri, E. (1979) *Textbook of Imported Diseases.* Oxford: OUP.

Oakley, R. (1979) Family, Kinship and Patronage: The Cypriot migration to Britain. In V. Saifullah Khan (ed.) *Minority Families in Britain: Support and Stress.* London: Macmillan.

Oberg, K. (1954) *Culture Shock.* Indianapolis: Bobbs-Merrill.

Obeyesekere, J. (1969) The Idiom of Demonic Possession: A Case Study. Reviewed in *Transcultural Psychiatry Research Review* **VI**, April.

Ødegaard, O. (1932) Emigration and Insanity. Copenhagen Supplement No. 4 to *Acta Psychiatrica Neurologica.*

———— (1936) Emigration and Mental Health. *Mental Hygiene* **20**: 546-53. Reprinted in C. Zwingmann and M. Pfieffer-Ammende (eds) *Uprooting and After.* New York: Springer-Verlag.

———— (1945) Distribution of Mental Diseases in Norway. *Acta Psychiatrica Neurologica* **20**: 247–63.

Ortiz, S. (1971) Reflections on the Concept of Peasant Culture and Peasant Cognitive Systems. In T. Shanin (ed.) *Peasants and Peasant Societies.* Harmondsworth: Penguin.

Osborne, Noble, and Weyl (1978) (eds.) *Human Variation: The Biopsychology of Age, Race, and Sex.* New York: Academic Press.

Patterson, S. (1963) *Dark Strangers.* London: Tavistock.

Parekh, B. (1974) The Spectre of Self-consciousness. In Pareth (ed.) *Colour, Culture, and Consciousness.* London: George Allen and Unwin.

Park, R. (1928) Human Migration and the Marginal Man. *American Journal of Sociology* **XXXIII**(6): 881–93. Reprinted in J. Stone (1977) *Race, Ethnicity and Social Change.* North Scituate, Mass.: Duxbury Press.

Pennsylvania Department of Public Welfare (1979) *National Mental Health Needs Assessment of Indo-Chinese Refugee Populations.* Bureau of Research and Training, Office of Mental Health.

Petersen, W. (1958) A General Typology of Migration *American Sociological Review* **23**.

Pfeiffer, W. M. (1968) The Symptomatology of Depression Viewed Transculturally. *Transcultural Psychiatry Research Review* **V**: 121–24.

Phillips, S. and Pearson, R. J. (1981) Practice Research dealing with Vietnamese Refugees. *British Medical Journal* **282**.

Philpott, S. B. (1977) The Montserratians: Migration Dependency and the Maintenance of Island Ties in England. In J. L. Watson (ed.) *Between Two Cultures.* Oxford: Blackwell.

Pinsent, R. F. N. (1963) Morbidity in an Immigrant Population. *Lancet* **I**: 437–38.

Pinto, R. (1974a) Psychosocial Variables Associated with Mental Illness in Patients of Asian Origin. *Indian Journal of Psychiatry* **16**: 197–202.

—— (1974b) A Comparison of Illness Patterns in Asian and English Patients. *Indian Journal of Psychiatry* **16**:203–10.

Power, J. in collaboration with A. Hardman (1976) Western Europe's Migrant Workers. Minority Rights Group Report No. 28. London: MRG (revised 1978).

Prange, A. J. (1959) An Interpretation of Cultural Isolation and Aliens' Paranoid Reaction. *International Journal of Social Psychiatry* **4**: 254–64.

Price, G. (1967) Mental Health Problems in Pre-School West Indian Children. *Maternal Child Care*, June: 483–86.

Price, J. (1975) Foreign Language Interpreting in Psychiatric Practice. *Australian and New Zealand Journal of Psychiatry* **9**: 263.

Rack, P. H. (1977) Some Practical Problems in Providing a Psychiatric Service for Immigrants. *Mental Health and Society* **4**: 144–51.

—— (1978) Immigrant Families and the Health Service. In *Off to a Good Start.* London: National Association for Maternal and Child Welfare.

—— (1979) Diagnosing Mental Illness: Asians and the Psychiatric Services. In V. Saifullah Khan (ed.) *Minority Families in Britain: Support and Stress.* London: Macmillan.

—— (1980) Ethnic Differences in Depression and its Response to Treatment. *Journal of International Medical Research*, Supplement (3): 20–23.

—— (1981) Aftermath of Empire: Pakistanis in Britain. In L. Eitinger and D. Schwarz (eds.) *Strangers in the World*. Bern: Hans Huber.

—— (1982) Migration and Mental Illness: A Review of Recent Research in Britain. *Transcultural Psychiatry Research Review* **xix** (3): 151–72.

Rahe, R. H., Looney, J. G., Ward, H. W., Tung, Tran Mina, and Liv, W. T. (1978) Psychiatric Consultation in a Vietnamese Refugee Camp. *American Journal of Psychiatry* **135**(2): 185–90.

Rahman, R. (1970) Depression — A Preliminary Review of 31 Patients (unpublished). Reviewed in *Transcultural Psychiatric Research Review* **29**.

Rao, A. V. (1966) Depression — A Psychiatric Analysis of Thirty Cases. *Indian Journal of Psychiatry* **8**(2): 143–54.

—— (1973) Depressive Illness and Guilt in Indian Culture. *Indian Journal of Psychiatry* **15**: 231–36.

Raskin, A. and Crook, T. (1975) Antidepressants in Black and White In-Patients. Differential Response to a Controlled Trial in Chlorpromazine and Imipramine. *Archives of General Psychiatry* **32**: 643.

Rendon, M. (1976) Transcultural Aspects of Mental Illness among Puerto Rican Adolescents in New York. In E. Fuchs (ed.) *Youth in a Changing World: Cross-Cultural Perspectives on Adolescence*. The Hague: Mouton.

Rex, J. (1973) *Race, Colonialism and the City*. London: Routledge and Kegan Paul.

Richie, J. (1964) Using an Interpreter Effectively. *Nursing Outlook* (December) **12**: 27–29.

Risso, M. and Böker, W. (1974) *Delusions of Bewitchment* Bibl. Psychiat. Neurol. Fasc. 124. Basel: Narger 1974. Summarized in C. Zwingmann, 1977.

Rogers, E. M. and Shoemaker, F. F. (1974) *Communication of Innovation*. New York: The Free Press/Macmillan.

Roskies, E. (1978) Immigration and Mental Health. *Canada's Mental Health* **26**(2): 4–6.

Rowell, V. and Rack, P. H. (1979) Health Education Needs of a Minority Ethnic Group. *Journal of the Institute of Health Education* **17**: 4.

Royer, J. (1977) *Black Britain's Dilemma: A Medico-Social Transcultural Study of West Indians*. Roseau, Dominica: Tropical Printers Ltd.

Runnymede Trust (n.d.) *Ethnic Minorities in Britain: A Select Bibliography*. London: Runnymede Trust.

Rutter, M., Yule, W., and Berger, M. (1974) The Children of West Indian Migrants. *New Society*, 14 March.

Rutter, M., Yule, B., Berger, M., Yule, N., Morton, J., and Bagley, C.

(1974) Children of West Indian Immigrants I. Rates of Behavioural Deviance and of Psychiatric Disorder. *Journal of Child Psychology and Psychiatry* **15**: 241–62.

Rwegellera, G. G. C. (1977) Psychiatric Morbidity among West Africans and West Indians Living in London. *Psychological Medicine* **7**: 317.

——— (1980) Differential Use of Psychiatric Services by West Indians, West Africans and English in London. *British Journal of Psychiatry* **137**: 428.

Saifullah Khan, V. (1974) 'Pakistani Villagers in a British City.' University of Bradford, Ph.D. Thesis (unpublished).

——— (1975) Asian Women in Britain: Strategies of Adjustment of Indian and Pakistani Migrants. In A. de Souza (ed.) *Women in Contemporary India.* Delhi: Mandhar.

——— (1976a) Purdah in the British Situation. In D. C. Barker and S. Allen (eds.) *Dependence and Exploitation in Work and Marriage.* London: Longmans.

——— (1976b) Pakistani Women in Britain. *New Community* **5**.

——— (1977) The Pakistanis: Mirpuri Villagers at Home and in the City of Bradford. In J. L. Watson (ed.) *Between Two Cultures.* Oxford: Blackwell.

——— (1979) (ed.) *Minority Families in Britain: Support and Stress.* London: Macmillan.

Sanua, V. D. (1969) Immigration, Migration and Mental Illness: A Review of the Literature with Special Emphasis on Schizophrenia. In E. B. Brady (ed.) *Behaviour in New Environments.* Beverley Hills: Sage Publications.

Sargant, W. (1973) *The Mind Possessed.* London: Heinemann.

Sartre, J.-P. (1957) Introduction to A. Memmi *Portrait du Colonisé Précedé du Portrait du Colonisateur.* Corrêa: Buchet/Chastel. English translation by H. Greenfield, published as *The Coloniser and the Colonised.* British Edition 1974, London: Souvenir Press.

Sashidharan, S. P. (1981) South Africa and the Royal College of Psychiatrists. *Lancet*: 1049.

Scarman, Rt. Hon. the Lord (1981) *The Brixton Disorders 10–12 April 1981* London: HMSO, Cmnd 8427.

Schlicht, J. and Carmichael, C. (1976) *Aspects of Mental Health in a Multi-cultural Society: Notes for the Guidance of Doctors and Social Workers.* London: Commission for Racial Equality.

Schneider, K. (1959) *Clinical Psychopathology.* New York: Orme and Stratton.

Schumacher, E. F. (1974) *Small is Beautiful.* London: Abacus (Sphere Books).

Sedlak, V. (1977) Community Psychiatry: A Rationale and an Illustration. Thesis for M.Sc. University of Leeds 1977.

Selvon, S. (1956) *The Lonely Londoners.* London. Longman Drumbeat.

Shaikh, A. and Bhate, S. (1980) *How Asian Patients Compare with Indigenous Patients in Leicestershire.* Transcultural Psychiatry Society (UK) Workshop, Leicester October 1980 (unpublished).

Simpson, G. E. and Yinger, J. M. (1953) *Racial and Cultural Minorities: An Analysis of Prejudice and Discrimination.* New York: Harper and Row.

Sims, A. C. P. and Symonds, R. C. (1975) Psychiatric Referrals from the Police. *British Journal of Psychiatry* **127**: 171–79.

Smith, D. J. (1977) *Racial Disadvantage in Britain.* The PEP Report. Harmondsworth: Penguin.

Smith, N. J. and McCulloch, J. W. (1976) Immigrants' Knowledge and Experience of Social Work Services. Paper read at International Congress on Transcultural Psychiatry. University of Bradford. (Unpublished.)

Spradley, J. P. and McCurdy, D. W. (1974) Editors' introduction to *Conformity and Conflict: Readings in Cultural Anthropology.* Boston: Little, Brown.

Stein, B. (1980) The Refugee Experience: An Overview of Refugee Research. Michigan State University, February 1980. (Unpublished.)

Stoller, A. (1981) Foreigners in Our Time (2). In L. Eitinger and D. Schwarz (eds) *Strangers in the World.* Bern: Hans Huber.

Stoneqvist, E. V. (1937) *The Marginal Man.* New York: Russell and Russell (reissued 1961).

Szasz, T. S. (1961) *The Myth of Mental Illness.* New York: Hoeber-Harper.

——— (1971) *The Manufacture of Madness.* London: Routledge and Kegan Paul.

Tajfel, H. (1978) *The Social Psychology of Minorities.* (MRG Report No. 38) London: Minority Rights Group.

Tannahill, J. A. (1958) *European Volunteer Workers.* Manchester: Manchester University Press.

Taylor, J. H. (1976) *The Halfway Generation.* Windsor: Berks. NFER Publishing Co.

Tewfik, G. I. and Okasha, A. (1965) *Psychosis and Immigration.* Postgraduate Medical Journal **41**: 603–12.

Thomas, W. I. and Znaniecki, F. (1918) *The Polish Peasant in Europe and America.* New York: Dover Publications (reprinted 1958).

Thompson, M. (1974) The Second Generation: Punjabi or English? *New Community* **III**(3): 242–48.

Toffler, A. (1970) *Future Shock.* London: Pan Books.

Tones, K. (1977) Communication of Innovations Theory. Notes for M. Phil students, Leeds Polytechnic.

Tonks, C. M., Paybel, E. S., and Klerman, G. L. (1970) Clinical Depressions among Negroes. *American Journal of Psychiatry* **127**(3).

Torrey, F. (1972) *The Mind Game: Witchdoctors and Psychiatrists.* New York: Emmerson.

—— (1974) *The Death of Psychiatry.* New York: Penguin Books.

Tyhurst, L. (1951) Displacement and Migration. *American Journal of Psychiatry* **107**: 561–68.

—— (1977) Psychosocial First Aid for Refugees: An Essay in Social Psychiatry. *Mental Health and Society* **4**: 319–43.

Tyler, E. B. (1874) *Primitive Culture: Researches into the Development of Mythology, Philosophy, Religion, Language, Art and Custom.* Reprinted 1958 as *The Origins of Culture.* New York: Harper and Row.

UNESCO (1952) *Statement on the Nature of Race and Race Differences.* Conference of Physical Anthropologists and Geneticists, September 1952. UNESCO.

Vasquez, A. (1980) Adolescents from the Southern Core of Latin America in Exile: Some Psychological Problems. In *Mental Health and Exile* (1981), WUS.

Wakil, P. A. (1970) Explorations of the Kin Networks of the Punjabi Society. *Journal of Marriage and the Family* **70**: 700–707.

Walker, I. M., Aslam, M., and Davis, S. S. (1980) Use of a Bradford Pharmacy by the Asian and Indigenous Population. *Pharmacological Journal* 20–27 December.

Wallace, A. F. C. (1961) *Culture and Personality.* New York: Random House.

Wandsworth Council for Community Relations (1978) *Asians and the Health Service: A Directory of Measures implemented by Area Health Authorities to Meet the Needs of the Asian Community.* WCRC, June.

Watson, J. L. (ed.) (1977) *Between Two Cultures: Migrants and Minorities in Britain.* Oxford: Blackwell.

Weinreich, P. (1975) Identity Diffusion in Immigrant and English Adolescents. In G. K. Verma and C. Bagley (eds) *Race Education and Identity.* London: Macmillan.

—— (1977) *Cultural Differences in Adolescent Identity Conflicts.* Vancouver: WFMH Congress (unpublished).

—— (1979) Ethnicity and Adolescent Identity Conflicts. In V. Saifullah Khan *Minority Families in Britain.* London: Macmillan.

Wellman, D. T. (1977) *Portraits of White Racism.* London: Cambridge University Press.

West Yorkshire Language Link (1978) The Background of Asian Patients.

Pilot Course at Staincliffe Hospital, Dewsbury: Post Course Evaluation Report. (Unpublished.)

Whitford, G. M. (1978) Acetylator Status in Relation to Monoamine Oxidase Antidepressant Drug Therapy. Presented at the International Congress of Transcultural Psychiatry, Bradford. *International Pharmacopsychiatry* **13**: 126–32.

Williams, E. (1961) Massa Day Done. Reprinted in D. Lowenthal and L. Comitas (eds) *The Aftermath of Sovereignty: West Indian Perspectives.* New York: Anchor Press/Doubleday.

Williams, W. M. (1956) *The Sociology of an English Village: Gosforth.* London: Routledge and Kegan Paul.

Wilson, Amrit (1978) *Finding a Voice: Asian Women in Britain.* London: Virago.

—— (1981) *Black People and the Health Service.* Brent Community Health Council, April.

Winokur, G., Clayton, P. J., and Reich, T. (1969) *Manic Depressive Illness.* St Louis: C. V. Mosby Co.

Wiser, C. V. and Wiser, W. H. (1951) *Behind Mud Walls.* New York: Agricultural Missions Inc. (Quotations are taken from G. M. Foster (1967).)

World Health Organisation (1972) *The International Pilot Study of Schizophrenia.* Geneva: WHO.

—— (1977) *Apartheid and Mental Health Care.* Report prepared for UN Special Committee against Apartheid MNH/775.

World University Service (1979) *Seminar on Mental Health and Exile: Chile.* London: WUS.

—— (1981) *Mental Health and Exile.* London WUS.

Yap, P. M. (1951) *Mental Diseases Peculiar to Certain Cultures.* Journal of Mental Science **97**: 313–27.

—— (1964) Suk-Yeon or Koro — A Culture-Bound Depersonalisation Syndrome. *Bulletin of the Hong Kong Chinese Medical Association* **16**(1): 31. Cited in Kiev (1972) *Transcultural Psychiatry.*

—— (1965) Affective Disorders in Chinese Culture in De Rueck and Porter (eds.) *Transcultural Psychiatry.* London: Churchill.

Zeigler, V. E. and Biggs, J. T. (1977) Tricyclic Plasma Levels. Effects of Age, Race, Sex and Smoking. *Journal of the American Medical Association* **238**: 2167.

Zubrzycki, T. (1956) *Polish Immigrants in Britain: A Study of Adjustment.* The Hague: Martinus Nijhoff.

Zwingmann, C. (1977) *Uprooting and Related Phenomena: A Descriptive Bibliography.* Geneva: WHO publication MNH/78. 23.

Zwingmann, C. and Pfister-Ammende, M. (1973) (eds) *Uprooting and After* New York: Springer-Verlag.

Name Index

Subject Index